ESSENTIAL PSYCHOPHARMACOLOGY OF ANTIPSYCHOTICS AND MOOD STABILIZERS

STEPHEN M. STAHL, M.D., Ph.D

University of California, San Diego
and Neuroscience Education Institute

With illustrations by
Nancy Muntner

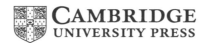

CAMBRIDGE
UNIVERSITY PRESS

PUBLISHED BY THE PRESS SYNDICATE OF THE UNIVERSITY OF CAMBRIDGE
The Pitt Building, Trumpington Street, Cambridge, United Kingdom

CAMBRIDGE UNIVERSITY PRESS
The Edinburgh Building, Cambridge CB2 2RU, UK
40 West 20th Street, New York, NY 10011-4211, USA
477 Williamstown Road, Port Melborne, VIC 3207, Australia
Ruiz de Alarcón 13, 28014 Madrid, Spain
Dock House, The Waterfront, Cape Town 8001, South Africa

http://www.cambridge.org

Every effort has been made in preparing this book to provide accurate and
up-to-date information that is in accord with accepted standards and practice
at the time of publication. Nevertheless, the authors, editors, and publisher
can make no warranties that the information contained herein is totally free
from error, not least because clinical standards are constantly changing
through research and regulation. The authors, editors, and publisher
therefore disclaim all liability for direct or consequential damages resulting
from the use of material contained in this book. Readers are strongly advised
to pay careful attention to information provided by the manufacturer of any
drugs that they plan to use.

First published 2002

Printed in the United States of America

Typeface Adobe Garamond 10/12 pts   *System* QuarkXPress™   [HT]

Library of Congress Cataloging in Publication Data is available

A catalog record for this book is available from the British Library

ISBN 0521 89074 8 paperback

Essential Psychopharmacology of Antipsychotics and Mood Stabilizers

Updated from the best-selling second edition of *Essential Psychopharmacology*, in this new book Stephen Stahl has revised the chapters covering antipsychotics and mood stabilizers. New material includes discussion of two new theories about dopaminergic modulation of receptors by new antipsychotic drugs: firstly, the "fast dissociation" (hit and run) hypothesis for how the atypical antipsychotics act, and secondly, a whole new class of antipsychotic agent, known as dopamine system stabilizers, with the prototypical agent aripiprazole. Also covered is the use of anti-convulsant agents to treat manic psychosis and the newest atypical antipsychotic ziprasidone. The antipsychotics chapter has increased by a third, with nearly fifty new images to illustrate the stunning advances in antipsychotic and mood stabilizer treatments since the publication of the second edition. This book will be essential reading for all professionals treating psychosis, and students who need to know the mechanisms of drug actions. CME self-assessment tests are included.

Reviews of *Essential Psychopharmacology*, First Edition

"Essential reading ... I would thoroughly recommend this book to anyone who works with psychotropic drugs – or who has the task of teaching others about them!"
American Journal of Psychiatry

"Firmly grounded in contemporary neuroscience ... an excellent and comprehensive account of the pharmacology of drugs currently used to treat psychiatric disorders."
Psychological Medicine

"This masterful production will benefit a broad spectrum of readers, from students to knowledgeable and experienced psychopharmacologists."
Psychiatric Times

"Finally, an elegant and beautiful psychopharmacology text written by a basic scientist who is also a clinician."
Journal of Clinical Psychiatry

Stephen M. Stahl is Adjunct Professor of Psychiatry at the University of California, San Diego. He has conducted numerous research projects awarded by the National Institute of Mental Health, the Veterans Administration, and the pharmaceutical industry. The author of more than 200 articles and chapters, Dr. Stahl is an internationally recognized clinician, researcher, and teacher in psychiatry with subspecialty expertise in psychopharmacology.

In memory of Daniel X. Freedman, mentor, colleague, and scientific father.

To Cindy, my wife, best friend and tireless supporter.

To Jennifer and Victoria, my daughters, for their patience and understanding of the demands of authorship.

PREFACE

This book is an update of the two chapters from the second edition of *Essential Psychopharmacology* that deal exclusively with psychosis, schizophrenia, and their treatment with antipsychotic drugs. The knowledge base of psychopharmacology for psychosis and schizophrenia has expanded considerably in the two years since the publication of the second edition of *Essential Psychopharmacology*, and this updated edition attempts to reflect these changes. In most developed countries, antipsychotics have become the highest value therapeutic market, not only for psychiatry, but for medical therapeutics in general. Since prescribers are rapidly expanding their utilization of the newer antipsychotics for the treatment of disorders other than psychosis, such as for the treatment of cognition in Alzheimer disease and for mood stabilization in bipolar disorders, it is particularly important to understand how the drugs categorized here as "antipsychotics" work.

Before discussing what the specific contents of this book have to offer in the area of psychosis and schizophrenia and antipsychotic drugs, it may be useful to point out that this text attempts to present the fundamentals of psychopharmacology in a simplified and readily readable format. Therefore, this material should aid the reader when consulting more sophisticated textbooks as well as the professional literature. The organization of the information here also applies principles of programmed learning for the reader, namely repetition and interaction, which has been shown to enhance retention.

Therefore, it is suggested that novices first approach this text by going through the material from beginning to end, reviewing only the color graphics and the legends for these graphics. Virtually everything covered in the text is also covered in the graphics and icons. Once having gone through all the color graphics in these chapters, it is recommended that the reader then go back to the beginning of the book and read the entire text, reviewing the graphics at the same time. Finally, after the text has been read, the entire book can be rapidly reviewed again merely by reexamining the various color graphics in the book. This use of the materials will aid in programmed learning by the use of repetition and interaction with visual learning through graphics. Hopefully, the visual concepts learned by reviewing the graphics will reinforce the written concepts learned from the text. For those of you who are already familiar with psychopharmacology, this book should provide a good review from beginning to end.

The text for this book has been written at a conceptual level rather than at a pragmatic level and includes ideas that are simplifications and rules. Thus, this is not a text for the sophisticated subspecialist in psychopharmacology. Another feature of this book is that it is not extensively referenced to original papers but rather to textbooks and reviews, including several written by the author.

Some of the specific information the reader can expect from this book in the first chapter includes an explanation of psychosis in general, and of the disorder schizophrenia in particular. The various dimensions of symptoms of schizophrenia are discussed as well as the hypotheses for the etiology of schizophrenia, including neurodevelopmental and neurodegenerative theories. Included is an extensive description of two neurotransmitter systems: dopamine and glutamate.

The use of antipsychotic drugs is covered in the second chapter. This includes the classical neuroleptics, more than a dozen agents also known as conventional antipsychotics, and the new so-called "atypical" antipsychotics, as well as a new class of antipsychotic agents termed dopamine system stabilizers. The conventional antipsychotics have been well known for decades, but are falling out of use as modern treatment shifts to the use of atypical antipsychotics. The atypical antipsychotics are rapidly expanding into therapeutic use throughout the world and include the original atypical antipsychotic clozapine, and the newer agents risperidone, olanzapine, quetiapine, and ziprasidone, as well as several other agents in clinical development. The major atypical antipsychotics are differentiated from each other as members of the same class that nevertheless can be distinguished by their efficacies in different symptom dimensions and their side effect profiles. The mechanisms of action of both conventional and atypical antipsychotics are explained here with icons and color graphics, including explanation of two new theories about dopaminergic modulation of receptors by antipsychotics. These include the concept of fast dissociation or "hit and run" actions of atypical antipsychotics on dopamine receptors by atypical antipsychotics, as well as the introduction of a new class of antipsychotic agent, the dopamine system stabilizers, with the prototype aripiprazole. Also examined is the use of anticonvulsant agents as treatments for mania and as adjuncts to the treatment of psychosis and schizophrenia with antipsychotics. Finally, drug metabolism by the cytochrome P450 system and the interaction of these drugs with cholinergic, dopaminergic, and serotonergic neuronal systems are covered.

Best wishes for your first step on your journey into this fascinating field of psychopharmacology.

STEPHEN M. STAHL

CONTENTS

CHAPTER 1

PSYCHOSIS AND SCHIZOPHRENIA

Psychosis is a difficult term to define and is frequently misused, not only in the newspapers and movies and on television, but unfortunately among mental health professionals as well. Stigma and fear surround the concept of psychosis and the

Table 1–1. *Disorders in which psychosis is a defining feature*

Schizophrenia
Substance-induced (i.e., drug-induced) psychotic disorders
Schizophreniform disorder
Schizoaffective disorder
Delusional disorder
Brief psychotic disorder
Shared psychotic disorder
Psychotic disorder due to a general medical condition

average citizen worries about long-standing myths of "mental illness," including "psychotic killers," "psychotic rage," and the equivalence of "psychotic" with the pejorative term "crazy."

There is perhaps no area of psychiatry where misconceptions are greater than in the area of psychotic illnesses. The reader is well served to develop an expertise on the facts about the diagnosis and treatment of psychotic illnesses in order to dispel unwarranted beliefs and to help destigmatize this devastating group of illnesses. This chapter is not intended to list the diagnostic criteria for all the different mental disorders in which psychosis is either a defining feature or an associated feature. The reader is referred to standard reference sources (DSM-IV and ICD-10) for that information. Although schizophrenia will be emphasized here, we will approach psychosis as a syndrome associated with a variety of illnesses which are all targets for antipsychotic drug treatment.

Clinical Description of Psychosis

Psychosis is a syndrome, which is a mixture of symptoms that can be associated with many different psychiatric disorders but is not a specific disorder itself in diagnostic schemes such as DSM-IV or ICD-10. At a minimum, psychosis means delusions and hallucinations. It generally also includes symptoms such as disorganized speech, disorganized behavior, and gross distortions of reality testing.

Therefore, psychosis can be considered to be a set of symptoms in which a person's mental capacity, affective response, and capacity to recognize reality, communicate, and relate to others are impaired. Psychotic disorders have psychotic symptoms as their defining features, but there are other disorders in which psychotic symptoms may be present but are not necessary for the diagnosis.

Those *disorders that require the presence of psychosis* (Table 1–1) as a *defining* feature of the diagnosis include schizophrenia, substance-induced (i.e., drug-induced) psychotic disorder, schizophreniform disorder, schizoaffective disorder, delusional disorder, brief psychotic disorder, shared psychotic disorder, and psychotic disorder due to a general medical condition. *Disorders that may or may not have psychotic symptoms* (Table 1–2) as an *associated* feature include mania and depression as well as several cognitive disorders such as Alzheimer's dementia.

Psychosis itself can be paranoid, disorganized-excited, or depressive. Perceptual distortions and motor disturbances can be associated with any type of psychosis.

Table 1–2. *Disorders in which psychosis is an associated feature*

Mania
Depression
Cognitive disorders
Alzheimer dementia

Perceptual distortions include being distressed by hallucinatory voices; hearing voices that accuse, blame, or threaten punishment; seeing visions; reporting hallucinations of touch, taste, or odor; or reporting that familiar things and people seem changed. *Motor disturbances* are peculiar, rigid postures; overt signs of tension; inappropriate grins or giggles; peculiar repetitive gestures; talking, muttering, or mumbling to oneself; or glancing around as if hearing voices.

Paranoid Psychosis

In paranoid psychosis, the patient has paranoid projections, hostile belligerence, and grandiose expansiveness. *Paranoid projection* includes preoccupation with delusional beliefs; believing that people are talking about oneself; believing one is being persecuted or conspired against; and believing people or external forces control one's actions. *Hostile belligerence* is verbal expression of feelings of hostility; expressing an attitude of disdain; manifesting a hostile, sullen attitude; manifesting irritability and grouchiness; tending to blame others for problems; expressing feelings of resentment; and complaining and finding fault, as well as expressing suspicion of people. *Grandiose expansiveness* is exhibiting an attitude of superiority; hearing voices that praise and extol; and believing one has unusual powers, is a well-known personality, or has a divine mission.

Disorganized-Excited Psychosis

In a disorganized-excited psychosis, there is conceptual disorganization, disorientation, and excitement. *Conceptual disorganization* can be characterized by giving answers that are irrelevant or incoherent; drifting off the subject; using neologisms; or repeating certain words or phrases. *Disorientation* is not knowing where one is, the season of the year, the calendar year, or one's own age. *Excitement* is expressing feelings without restraint; manifesting hurried speech; exhibiting an elevated mood or an attitude of superiority; dramatizing oneself or one's symptoms; manifesting loud and boisterous speech; exhibiting overactivity or restlessness; and exhibiting excess of speech.

Depressive Psychosis

Depressive psychosis is characterized by retardation, apathy, and anxious self-punishment and blame. *Retardation and apathy* are manifested by slowed speech; indifference to one's future; fixed facial expression; slowed movements; deficiencies in recent memory; blocking in speech; apathy toward oneself or one's problems; slovenly appearance; low or whispered speech; and failure to answer questions. *Anxious self-punishment and blame* involve the tendency to blame or condemn oneself; anxiety about specific matters; apprehensiveness regarding vague future events; an attitude of self-deprecation; manifesting a depressed mood; expressing feelings of guilt and remorse; preoccupation with suicidal thoughts, unwanted ideas, and specific fears; and feeling unworthy or sinful.

This discussion of clusters of psychotic symptoms does not constitute diagnostic criteria for any psychotic disorder. It is given merely as a description of several types of symptoms in psychosis to give the reader an overview of the nature of behavioral disturbances associated with the various psychotic illnesses.

Five Symptom Dimensions in Schizophrenia

Although schizophrenia is the most common and best known psychotic illness, it is not synonymous with psychosis but is just one of many causes of psychosis. Schizophrenia affects 1% of the population, and in the United States there are over 300,000 acute schizophrenic episodes annually. Between 25 and 50% of schizophrenia patients attempt suicide, and 10% eventually succeed, contributing to a mortality rate eight times as high as that of the general population. In the United States over 20% of all Social Security benefit days are used for the care of schizophrenic patients. The direct and indirect costs of schizophrenia in the United States alone are estimated to be in the tens of billions of dollars every year.

Schizophrenia by definition is a disturbance that must last for six months or longer, including at least one month of delusions, hallucinations, disorganized speech, grossly disorganized or catatonic behavior, or negative symptoms. *Delusions* usually involve a misinterpretation of perceptions or experiences. The most common type of delusion in schizophrenia is persecutory, but the delusions may include a variety of other themes, including referential (i.e., erroneously thinking that something refers to oneself), somatic, religious, or grandiose. *Hallucinations* may occur in any sensory modality (e.g., auditory, visual, olfactory, gustatory, and tactile), but auditory hallucinations are by far the most common and characteristic hallucinations in schizophrenia.

Although not recognized formally as part of the diagnostic criteria for schizophrenia, numerous studies subcategorize the symptoms of this illness (as well as symptoms of some other disorders) into five dimensions: positive symptoms, negative symptoms, cognitive symptoms, aggressive/hostile symptoms, and depressive/anxious symptoms (Fig. 1–1). Several illnesses other than schizophrenia share these symptoms dimensions as well (Figs. 1–2 to 1–6).

Positive Symptoms

Positive symptoms seem to reflect an *excess* of normal functions (Table 1–3) and typically include delusions and hallucinations; they may also include distortions or exaggerations in language and communication (disorganized speech), as well as in behavioral monitoring (grossly disorganized or catatonic or agitated behavior).

Disorders in addition to schizophrenia that can have positive symptoms include bipolar disorder, schizoaffective disorder, psychotic depression, Alzheimer's disease

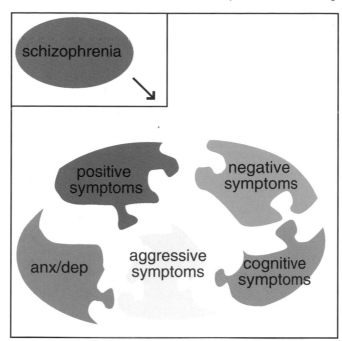

FIGURE 1–1. The **five symptom dimensions** of schizophrenia include not only positive and negative symptoms but also cognitive symptoms, aggressive/hostile symptoms, and depressive and anxious symptoms (anx/dep).

and other organic dementias, childhood psychotic illnesses, drug induced psychoses, and others (Fig. 1–2).

Negative Symptoms

Negative symptoms (Table 1–4) include at least five types of symptoms (all starting with the letter *a*): (1) *affective flattening*, consisting of restrictions in the range and intensity of emotional expression; (2) *alogia*, consisting of restrictions in the fluency and productivity of thought and speech; (3) *avolition*, consisting of restrictions in the initiation of goal-directed behavior; (4) *anhedonia*, that is, lack of pleasure; and (5) *attentional impairment*.

Negative symptoms commonly are considered a *reduction* in normal functions in schizophrenia, such as blunted affect, emotional withdrawal, poor rapport, passivity, and apathetic social withdrawal. Difficulty in abstract thinking, stereotyped thinking, and lack of spontaneity are associated with long periods of hospitalization and poor social functioning.

Negative symptoms in schizophrenia can be either primary or secondary (Fig. 1–3). Primary negative symptoms are considered to be those that are core to primary deficits of schizophrenia itself. Other core deficits of schizophrenia that may manifest themselves as negative symptoms may be those associated with or thought to be secondary to the positive symptoms of psychosis. Other negative symptoms are considered to be secondary to extrapyramidal symptoms (EPS), especially those

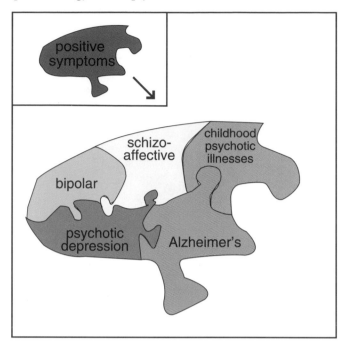

FIGURE 1–2. **Positive symptoms** are associated not just with schizophrenia, but also with bipolar disorder, schizoaffective disorder, childhood psychotic illnesses, psychotic depression, Alzheimer's disease, and other disorders as well.

caused by antipsychotic drugs. Negative symptoms can also be secondary to depressive symptoms or to environmental deprivation.

Cognitive Symptoms

Cognitive symptoms of schizophrenia and other illnesses of which psychosis may be an associated feature can overlap with negative symptoms. They include specifically the thought disorder of schizophrenia and the sometimes odd use of language, including incoherence, loose associations, and neologisms. Impaired attention and impaired information processing are other specific cognitive impairments associated with schizophrenia. In fact, the most common and the most severe of the cognitive impairments in schizophrenia can include impaired verbal fluency (ability to produce spontaneous speech), problems with serial learning (of a list of items or a sequence of events), and impairment in vigilance for executive functioning (problems with sustaining and focusing attention, concentrating, prioritizing, and modulating behavior based on social cues).

Schizophrenia is certainly not the only disorder with such impairments in cognition. Autism, poststroke dementia, Alzheimer's disease, and many other organic dementias (parkinsonian/Lewy body dementia, frontotemporal/Pick's dementia, etc.) are also associated with some cognitive dysfunctions similar to those seen in schizophrenia (Fig. 1–4).

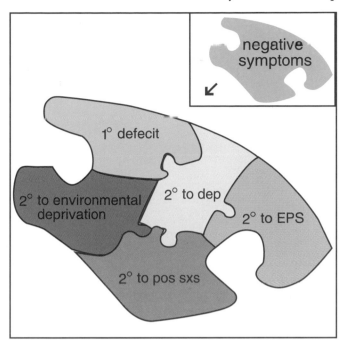

FIGURE 1–3. **Negative symptoms** in schizophrenia can either be a primary deficit of the illness (1° deficit) or secondary to depression (2° to dep), secondary to extrapyramidal symptoms (2° to EPS), secondary to environmental deprivation, or even secondary to positive symptoms (2° to pos sxs) in schizophrenia.

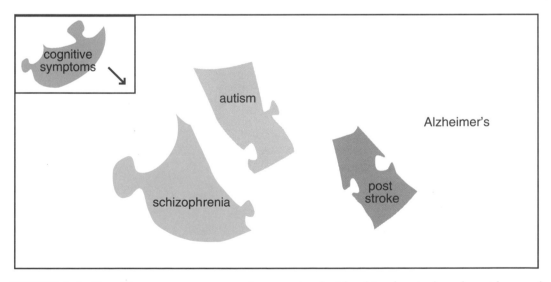

FIGURE 1–4. **Cognitive symptoms** are not just associated with schizophrenia, but also with several other disorders, including autism, Alzheimer's disease, and conditions following cerebrovascular accidents (poststroke).

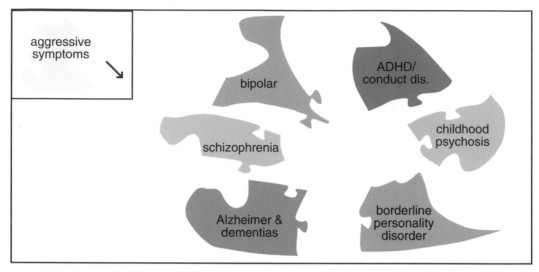

FIGURE 1–5. **Aggressive symptoms and hostility** are associated with several conditions in addition to schizophrenia, including bipolar disorder, attention deficit hyperactivity disorder (ADHD) and conduct disorder (conduct dis.), childhood psychosis, Alzheimer's and other dementias, and borderline personality disorder, among others.

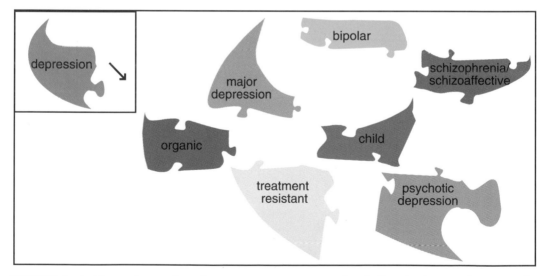

FIGURE 1–6. **Depressive and anxious symptoms** are not only a hallmark of major depressive disorder but are frequently associated with other psychiatric disorders, including bipolar disorder, schizophrenia, and schizoaffective disorder; with organic causes of depression, such as substance abuse; with childhood mood disorders (child); with psychotic forms of depression; and with mood and psychotic disorders resistant to treatment with drugs (treatment-resistant), among others.

Table 1–3. *Positive symptoms of psychosis*

Delusions
Hallucinations
Distortions or exaggerations in language and communication
Disorganized speech
Disorganized behavior
Catatonic behavior
Agitation

Table 1–4. *Negative symptoms of psychosis*

Blunted affect
Emotional withdrawal
Poor rapport
Passivity
Apathetic social withdrawal
Difficulty in abstract thinking
Lack of spontaneity
Stereotyped thinking
Alogia: restrictions in fluency and productivity of thought and speech
Avolition: restrictions in initiation of goal-directed behavior
Anhedonia: lack of pleasure
Attentional impairment

Aggressive and Hostile Symptoms

Aggressive and hostile symptoms can overlap with positive symptoms but specifically emphasize problems in impulse control. They include overt hostility, such as verbal or physical abusiveness or even assault. Such symptoms also include self-injurious behaviors, including suicide and arson or other property damage. Other types of impulsiveness, such as sexual acting out, are also in this category of aggressive and hostile symptoms.

Although aggressive symptoms are common in schizophrenia, they are far from unique to this condition. Thus, these same symptoms are frequently associated with bipolar disorder, childhood psychosis, borderline personality disorder, drug abuse, Alzheimer and other dementias, attention deficit hyperactivity disorder, conduct disorders in children, and many others (Fig. 1–5).

Depressive and Anxious Symptoms

Depressive and anxious symptoms are frequently associated with schizophrenia, but this does not necessarily mean that they fulfill the diagnostic criteria for a comorbid anxiety or affective disorder. Nevertheless, depressed mood, anxious mood, guilt, tension, irritability, and worry frequently accompany schizophrenia. These various symptoms are also prominent features of major depressive disorder, psychotic depression, bipolar disorder, schizoaffective disorder, organic dementias, and childhood psychotic disorders, among others, and particularly of treatment-resistant cases of depression, bipolar disorder, and schizophrenia (Fig. 1–6).

Four Key Dopamine Pathways and the Biological Basis of Schizophrenia

The biological basis of schizophrenia remains unknown. However, the monoamine neurotransmitter dopamine has played a key role in hypotheses about certain aspects of the five dimensions of symptoms in schizophrenia, discussed above.

Four well-defined dopamine pathways in the brain are shown in Figure 1–7. They include the mesolimbic dopamine pathway, the mesocortical dopamine pathway, the nigrostriatal dopamine pathway, and the tuberoinfundibular dopamine pathway.

Mesolimbic Dopamine Pathway and the Dopamine Hypothesis of the Positive Symptoms of Psychosis

The *mesolimbic dopamine pathway* projects from dopaminergic cell bodies in the ventral tegmental area of the brainstem to axon terminals in limbic areas of the brain, such as the nucleus accumbens (Fig. 1–8). This pathway is thought to have an important role in emotional behaviors, especially auditory hallucinations but also delusions and thought disorder (Fig. 1–9).

For more than 25 years, it has been observed that diseases or drugs that increase dopamine will enhance or produce positive psychotic symptoms, whereas drugs that decrease dopamine will decrease or stop positive symptoms. For example, stimulant drugs such as amphetamine and cocaine release dopamine and if given repetitively, can cause a paranoid psychosis virtually indistinguishable from schizophrenia. Also, all known antipsychotic drugs capable of treating positive psychotic symptoms are blockers of dopamine receptors, particularly D2 dopamine receptors. Antipsychotic drugs are discussed in Chapter 2. These observations have been formulated into a theory of psychosis sometimes referred to as the dopamine hypothesis of schizophrenia. Perhaps a more precise modern designation is the *mesolimbic dopamine hypothesis of positive psychotic symptoms*, since it is believed that it is hyperactivity specifically in this particular dopamine pathway that mediates the positive symptoms of psychosis (Fig. 1–9). Hyperactivity of the mesolimbic dopamine pathway hypothetically accounts for positive psychotic symptoms whether those symptoms are part of the illness of schizophrenia or of drug-induced psychosis, or whether positive psychotic symptoms accompany mania, depression, or dementia. Hyperactivity of mesolimbic dopamine neurons may also play a role in aggressive and hostile symptoms in schizophrenia and related illnesses, especially if serotonergic control of dopamine is aberrant in patients who lack impulse control.

Mesocortical Dopamine Pathway

A pathway related to the mesolimbic dopamine pathway is the *mesocortical dopamine pathway* (Fig. 1–10). Its cell bodies arise in the ventral tegmental area of the brainstem, near the cell bodies for the dopamine neurons of the mesolimbic dopamine pathway. However, the mesocortical dopamine pathway projects to areas of the cerebral cortex, especially the limbic cortex. The role of the mesocortical dopamine

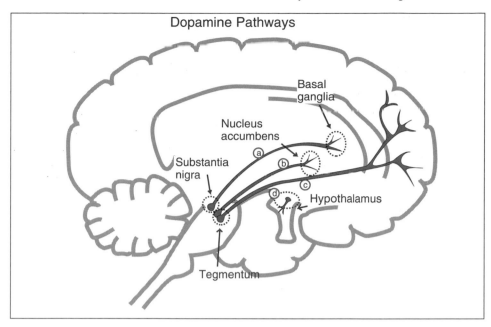

FIGURE 1–7. **Four dopamine pathways in the brain**. The neuroanatomy of dopamine neuronal pathways in the brain can explain both the therapeutic effects and the side effects of the known antipsychotic agents. (a) The **nigrostriatal dopamine pathway** projects from the substantia nigra to the basal ganglia, is part of the extrapyramidal nervous system, and controls movements. (b) The **mesolimbic dopamine pathway** projects from the midbrain ventral tegmental area to the nucleus accumbens, a part of the limbic system of the brain thought to be involved in many behaviors, such as pleasurable sensations, the powerful euphoria of drugs of abuse, as well as delusions and hallucinations of psychosis. (c) A pathway related to the mesolimbic dopamine pathway is the **mesocortical dopamine pathway**. It also projects from the midbrain ventral tegmental area, but sends its axons to the limbic cortex, where they may have a role in mediating negative and cognitive symptoms of schizophrenia. (d) The fourth dopamine pathway of interest controls prolactin secretion and is called the **tuberoinfundibular dopamine pathway**. It projects from the hypothalamus to the anterior pituitary gland.

pathway in mediating negative and/or cognitive symptoms of schizophrenia is still a matter of debate. Some researchers believe that negative symptoms and possibly certain cognitive symptoms of schizophrenia may be due to a deficit of dopamine in mesocortical projection areas, such as the *dorsolateral prefrontal cortex* (Figs. 1–10 and 1–11). The behavioral deficit state suggested by negative symptoms certainly implies underactivity or even "burnout" of neuronal systems. This may be related to excitotoxic overactivity of *glutamate systems*. An ongoing degenerative process in the mesocortical dopamine pathway could explain a progressive worsening of symptoms and an ever-increasing deficit state in some schizophrenic patients.

In this formulation of negative and cognitive symptoms of schizophrenia as a dopamine deficiency state of mesocortical dopamine neurons, the deficiency could hypothetically be either a primary dopamine deficit or a dopamine deficit secondary to inhibition by an excess of serotonin in this pathway (Fig. 1–11). The dopamine deficiency could also be secondary to blockage of dopamine 2 receptors

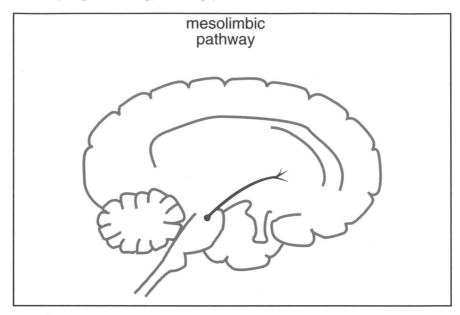

FIGURE 1–8. This diagram shows the **mesolimbic dopamine pathway**, which is thought to be hyperactive in schizophrenia and to mediate the **positive symptoms** of psychosis.

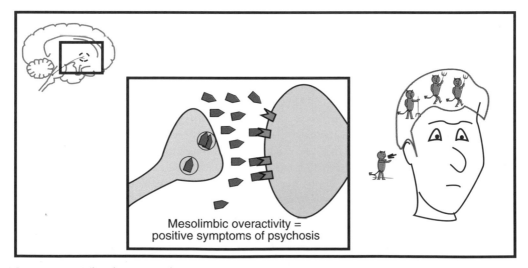

FIGURE 1–9. **The dopamine hypothesis of psychosis**. Hyperactivity of dopamine neurons in the mesolimbic dopamine pathway theoretically mediates the positive symptoms of psychosis, such as delusions and hallucinations. This pathway is also involved in pleasure, reward, and reinforcing behavior, and many drugs of abuse interact here.

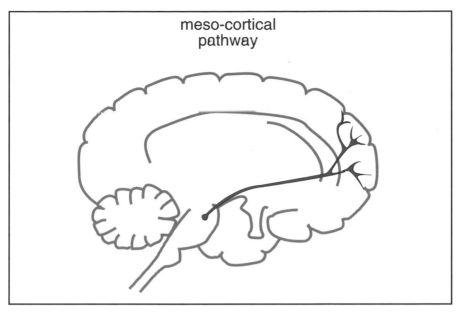

FIGURE 1–10. The **mesocortical dopamine pathway** mediates the negative and cognitive symptoms of psychosis.

by antipsychotic drugs. This will be discussed in greater detail in Chapter 2. Theoretically, increasing dopamine in the mesocortical dopamine pathway might improve negative symptoms or possibly even cognitive symptoms. However, since there is hypothetically already an excess of dopamine in the mesolimbic dopamine pathway, any further increase of dopamine in that pathway would actually worsen positive symptoms. Thus, this poses a therapeutic dilemma: How can one increase dopamine in the mesocortical pathway simultaneously with decreasing dopamine activity in the mesolimbic dopamine pathway? The extent to which atypical antipsychotics have provided a solution to this therapeutic dilemma will be discussed in Chapter 2.

Nigrostriatal Dopamine Pathway

Another key dopamine pathway in brain is the *nigrostriatal dopamine pathway*, which projects from dopaminergic cell bodies in the substantia nigra of the brainstem via axons terminating in the basal ganglia or striatum (Fig. 1–12). The nigrostriatal dopamine pathway is a part of the extrapyramidal nervous system and controls motor movements. Deficiencies in dopamine in this pathway cause movement disorders, including Parkinson's disease, which is characterized by rigidity, akinesia or bradykinesia (i.e., lack of movement or slowing of movement), and tremor. Dopamine deficiency in the basal ganglia also can produce akathisia (a type of restlessness) and dystonia (twisting movements, especially of the face and neck). These movement disorders which can be replicated by drugs that block dopamine 2 receptors in this pathway, will be discussed in Chapter 2.

Hyperactivity of dopamine in the nigrostriatal pathway is thought to underlie various hyperkinetic movement disorders, such as chorea, dyskinesias, and tics.

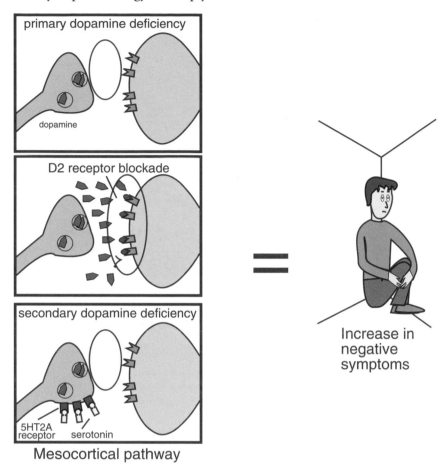

FIGURE 1–11. Several different causes of **dopamine deficiency** may result in **negative and cognitive symptoms**. In schizophrenia itself, there may be a primary dopamine (DA) deficiency or a DA deficiency secondary to blockade of postsynaptic D2 dopamine receptor by an antipsychotic drug. If serotonin is hyperactive, this may also cause a relative DA deficiency by inhibiting DA release. Either primary or secondary DA deficiency in this pathway may cause cognitive blunting, social isolation, indifference, apathy, and anhedonia.

Chronic blockade of dopamine 2 receptors in this pathway may result in a hyperkinetic movement disorder known as *neuroleptic-induced tardive dyskinesia*, which will be discussed further in Chapter 2.

Tuberoinfundibular Dopamine Pathway

The dopamine neurons that project from the hypothalamus to the anterior pituitary are known as the *tuberoinfundibular dopamine pathway* (Fig. 1–13). Normally, these neurons are active and *inhibit* prolactin release. In the postpartum state, however, their activity is decreased, and therefore prolactin levels can rise during breastfeeding, so that lactation will occur. If the functioning of tuberoinfundibular

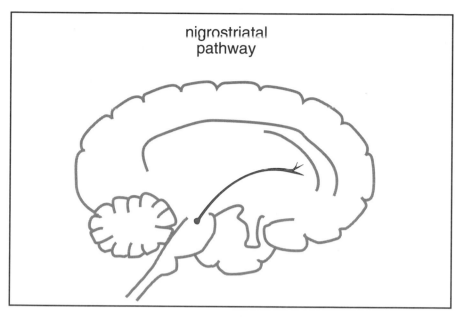

FIGURE 1–12. The **nigrostriatal dopamine pathway** is part of the extrapyramidal nervous system and plays a key role in regulating movements. When dopamine is deficient, it can cause parkinsonism with tremor, rigidity, and akinesia/bradykinesia. When DA is in excess, it can cause hyperkinetic movements such as tics and dyskinesias.

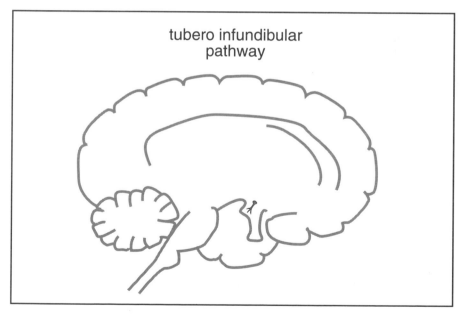

FIGURE 1–13. The **tuberoinfundibular** dopamine pathway from hypothalamus to anterior pituitary regulates prolactin secretion into the circulation. Dopamine inhibits prolactin secretion.

dopamine neurons is disrupted by lesions or drugs, prolactin levels can also rise. Elevated prolactin levels are associated with galactorrhea (breast secretions), amenorrhea, and possibly other problems, such as sexual dysfunction. Such problems can occur after treatment with many antipsychotic drugs that block dopamine 2 receptors, as will be discussed further in Chapter 2.

Neurodevelopmental Hypotheses of Schizophrenia

One leading hypothesis for the etiology of schizophrenia is that this illness originates from abnormalities in fetal brain development during the early stages of neuronal selection and migration. Although the symptoms of schizophrenia are usually not evident until the late teens to the twenties it may be that "the die is cast" much earlier. That is, an abnormal degenerative process may be "turned on" genetically very early in fetal brain development. However, symptoms do not occur until the brain extensively revises its synapses in adolescence, and it is hypothetically this normal restructuring process that unmasks the problems of neuronal selection and migration that were previously hidden. Although one idea is that the degenerative process may only do this type of fetal "hit and run" damage, it is also possible that the degenerative process continues during the symptomatic phase of schizophrenia, as discussed below in relation to the neurodegenerative hypothesis and combined neurodevelopmental/neurodegenerative hypothesis of schizophrenia.

Other support for the possibility that schizophrenia could have a neurodevelopmental basis includes observations that schizophrenia is increased in those with a fetal history of obstetric complications ranging from viral infections to starvation to autoimmune processes and other such problems in the pregnant mother. These observations suggest that an insult to the brain early in fetal development could contribute to the cause of schizophrenia. These risk factors may all have the final common pathway of reducing nerve growth factors, and also stimulating certain noxious processes that kill off critical neurons, such as cytokines, viral infection, hypoxia, trauma, starvation, or stress. This may be mediated either by apoptosis or by necrosis. The result (reviewed in Fig. 1–14) could be either overt structural abnormalities or more subtle problems, including selection of the wrong neurons to survive in the fetal brain, neuron migration to the wrong places, neuron innervation of the wrong targets, and mixup of the nurturing signals so that what innervates these neurons is also mixed up. Problems with proteins involved in the structural matrix of synapses (such as synapsins) may occur in schizophrenia, leading to reduced numbers of synaptic vesicles, aberrant synapse formation, and delays or reduction in synapse formation.

If schizophrenia is caused by abnormal early brain development (cf. Figs. 1–15 and 1–16), it may be virtually impossible to reverse such abnormalities in adulthood. On the other hand, some day it may be possible to compensate for such postulated neurodevelopmental difficulties by other mechanisms or to interrupt an ongoing mechanism still present in the symptomatic patient. Therefore, it will be critical to learn what neurodevelopmental abnormalities may exist in schizophrenia in order to devise strategies for reducing their potential impact. It may even be possible to identify such abnormalities in presymptomatic individuals or to exploit the plasticity of adult neurons to compensate for neurodevelopmentally endowed dysfunction. These are bold and unsubstantiated theoretical extrapolations based on

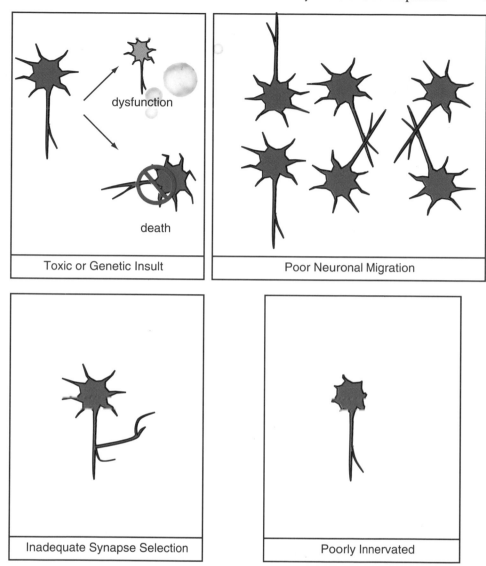

FIGURE 1–14. **Neurodevelopmental abnormalities** in schizophrenia may include toxic or genetic insults to neurons, either killing them or rendering their functioning inadequate; poor neuronal migration during fetal brain development; inadequate and improper selection of synaptic targets during synaptogenesis, especially before the age of 6; and/or inadequate innervation received from inputs of other neurons.

the most optimistic therapeutic visions; current molecular and neurodevelopmental approaches have not yet evolved into successful therapeutic strategies.

Strong evidence for a genetic basis of schizophrenia comes from twin studies. Scientists have been trying for a long time to identify abnormal genes in schizophrenia (Fig. 1–17) and the consequences that such abnormal genes could have on molecular regulation of neuronal functioning in schizophrenic patients (Fig. 1–18).

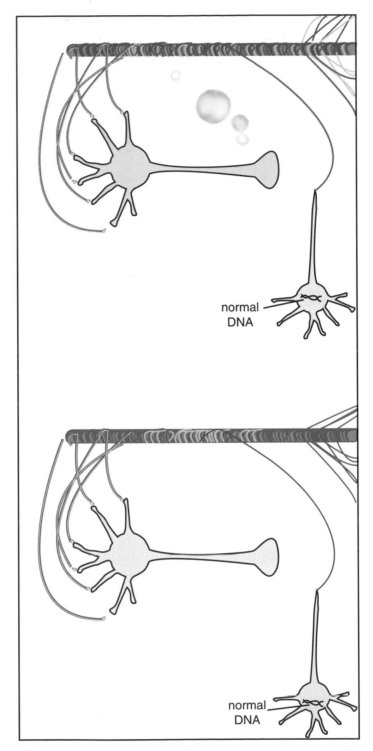

FIGURE 1–15. **Neurodevelopmental theories of schizophrenia** suggest that something goes wrong with the genetic program for the **normal formation of synapses and migration of neurons** in the brain during the prenatal and early childhood formation of the brain and its connections. Depicted here is a concept of how a neuron with normal genetic programming would develop and form synaptic connections.

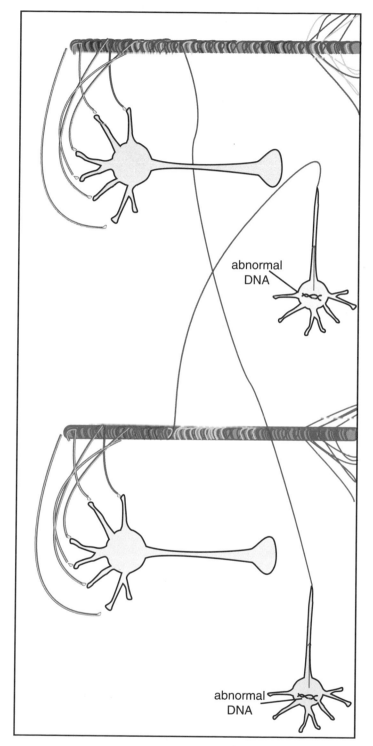

FIGURE 1–16. According to neurodevelopmental theories of schizophrenia, an abnormality in the DNA of a schizophrenic patient may cause the **wrong synaptic connections** to be made during the prenatal and early childhood formation of the brain and its connections. Schizophrenia may be the result of abnormal development of the brain from the beginning of life either because the wrong neurons are selected to survive into adulthood or because those neurons that do survive fail to migrate to the correct parts of the brain, fail to form appropriate connections, and then are subject to breakdown when put to use by the individual in late adolescence and adulthood.

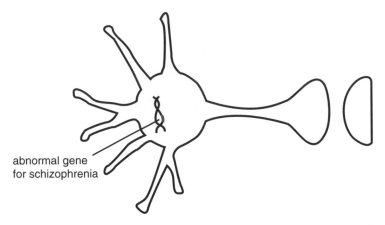

FIGURE 1–17. This figure shows one of the several **postulated abnormal genes** in schizophrenia that may contribute to the risk of this illness. Here it is lying dormant in the cell. In this case, it does not produce abnormal gene products or cause schizophrenia. Thus, it is not contributing to the risk of illness.

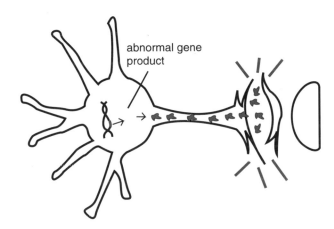

FIGURE 1–18. Here, the postulated **abnormal gene for schizophrenia** is being expressed, leading to an abnormal gene product that contributes to the risk of schizophrenia because it causes disruption in the functioning of the neuron. The manner of the disruption is additive with other risks from other genes and other environmental factors, with just the right timing and in just the right sequence; this, in turn, leads to psychosis and the other symptoms of schizophrenia.

It is already clear that the causes of psychotic illnesses such as schizophrenia and bipolar disorder are not going to be single abnormalities in a major genetic locus of DNA, like those already proven for diseases such as Huntington's disease. Rather, *multiple* genetic abnormalities are likely to *each* contribute in complex ways to a vulnerability to schizophrenia and other psychotic illnesses, perhaps only when other critical environmental inputs are also present. Thus, the genetic basis of schizophrenia is not likely to be as simple as depicted in Figures 1–17 and 1–18; rather, a whole list of abnormally acting genes and their corresponding gene products, triggered

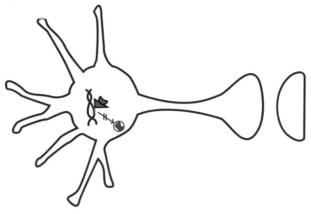

FIGURE 1–19. A highly theoretical direct **genetic approach to therapeutics** in schizophrenia is based on the notion that if dormant risk factors could be identified in the genome, perhaps drugs could prevent the expression of such genes and thus prevent the triggering of the disease process leading to schizophrenia.

from both inherited and acquired risk factors, are hypothesized to act together or in just the right sequence to cause the evolution of the symptom clusters known as schizophrenia. It will be important to determine just how these gene products participate in mediating the symptoms of schizophrenia, because only then could a logical biochemical rationale be found for preventing or interrupting these abnormalities by interfering with gene transcription, for example (Fig. 1–19), by blocking the action of unwanted gene products, or by substituting for the action of missing gene products. This is not likely to be simple, as multiple simultaneous drugs acting to compensate for each genetic abnormality might prove to be necessary, and treatments based on this approach do not appear to be imminent.

Neurodegenerative Hypotheses of Schizophrenia

The presence of both functional and structural abnormalities demonstrated in neuroimaging studies of the brain of schizophrenics suggests that a neurodegenerative process with progressive loss of neuronal function may be ongoing during the course of the disease. A neurodegenerative condition is also suggested by the progressive nature of the course of illness in schizophrenia (Fig. 1–20). Such a course of illness is not consistent with simply being the result of a static and previously completed pathological process.

Schizophrenia progresses from a largely asymptomatic stage prior to the teen years (phase I in Fig. 1–20), to a prodromal stage of "oddness" and the onset of subtle negative symptoms in the late teens to early twenties (phase II in Fig. 1–20). The active phase of the illness begins and continues throughout the twenties and thirties with destructive positive symptoms, characterized by an up-and-down course with treatment and relapse, with the patient never quite returning to the same level of functioning following acute relapses or exacerbations (phase III in Fig. 1–20). Finally, the disease can reach a largely stable level of poor social functioning and prominent negative and cognitive symptoms, with some ups and downs but at a

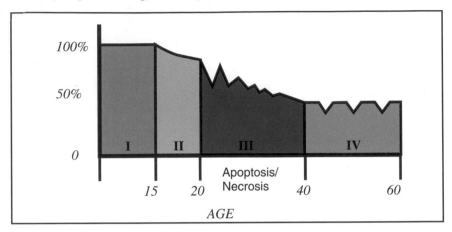

FIGURE 1–20. The **stages of schizophrenia** are shown here over a lifetime. The patient has full functioning (100%) early in life and is virtually asymptomatic (stage I). However, during a prodromal phase (stage II) starting in the teens, there may be odd behaviors and subtle negative symptoms. The acute phase of the illness usually announces itself fairly dramatically in the twenties (stage III), with positive symptoms, remissions, and relapses but never a complete return to previous levels of functioning. This is often a chaotic stage of the illness, with a progressive downhill course. The final phase of the illness (stage IV) may begin in the forties or later, with prominent negative and cognitive symptoms and some waxing and waning during its course, but often more of a burnout stage of continuing disability. There may not necessarily be a continuing and relentless downhill course, but the patient may become progressively resistant to treatment with antipsychotic medications during this stage.

considerable step-off from baseline functioning, suggesting a more static phase of illness sometimes called "burnout" in the forties or later in life (phase IV in Fig. 1–20).

The fact that a schizophrenic patient's responsiveness to antipsychotic treatment can change (and lessen) over the course of illness also suggests an ongoing neurodegenerative process of some kind. For example, the time it takes for a schizophrenic patient to go into remission increases in each successive psychotic relapse. A patient may be less responsive to antipsychotic treatment during successive episodes or exacerbations, so that residual symptoms remain as well as decrements in the patient's functional capacities. This development of treatment resistance during successive episodes of the illness suggests that "psychosis is hazardous to the brain." It thus seems possible that patients who receive early and effective continuous treatment may prevent disease progression or at least the development of treatment resistance.

Excitotoxicity

One major idea proposed to explain the downhill course of schizophrenia and the development of treatment resistance is that neurodegenerative events in schizophrenia may be mediated by a type of excessive action of the neurotransmitter glutamate that has come to be known as *excitotoxicity*. The excitotoxic hypothesis of schizophrenia proposes that neurons degenerate because of excessive excitatory neurotransmission at glutamate neurons. This process of excitotoxicity, not only is a hypothesis to explain neurodegeneration in schizophrenia but also has been invoked as an explanation for neurodegeneration in any number of neurological and psychiatric conditions, including Alzheimer's disease and other degenerative dementias, Parkinson's disease, amytrophic lateral sclerosis (Lou Gehrig's disease), and even stroke.

In order to understand the hypothesis of excessive excitation of neurons by glutamate, it is necessary to understand glutamatergic neurotransmission.

Glutamatergic Neurotransmission

Glutamate synthesis. The amino acid glutamate or glutamic acid is a neurotransmitter, but its predominant use is as an amino acid building block for protein biosynthesis. When used as a neurotransmitter, it is synthesized from glutamine (Fig. 1–21), which is converted to glutamate by an enzyme in mitochondria called *glutaminase*. It is then stored in synaptic vesicles for subsequent release during neurotransmission. Glutamine itself can be obtained from glial cells adjacent to neurons. The glial cells help to support neurons both structurally and metabolically. In the case of glutamate neurons, nearby glia can provide glutamine for neurotransmitter glutamate synthesis. In this case, glutamate from metabolic pools in the glia is converted into glutamate for use as a neurotransmitter. This is accomplished by first converting glutamate into glutamine in the glial cell via the enzyme glutamine synthetase. Glutamine is then transported into the neuron for conversion into glutamate for use as a neurotransmitter (Fig. 1–21).

Glutamate removal. Glutamate's actions are stopped not by enzymatic breakdown, as in other neurotransmitter systems, but by removal by two transport pumps. The first of these pumps is a presynaptic glutamate transporter, which works as do all the other neurotransmitter transporters already discussed for monoamine neurotransmitter systems such as dopamine, norepinephrine, and serotonin. The second transport pump, located on nearby glia, removes glutamate from the synapse and terminates its actions there. Glutamate removal is summarized in Figure 1–22.

Glutamate receptors. There are several types of glutamate receptors (Fig. 1–23), including N-methyl-*d*-asparate (NMDA), alpha-amino-3-hydroxy-5-methyl-4-isoxazole-propionic acid (AMPA), and kainate, all named after the agonists that selectively bind to them. Another type of glutamate receptor is the metabotropic glutamate receptor, which may mediate long-lasting electrical signals in the brain by a process called *long-term potentiation* which appears to have a key role in memory functions.

The NMDA, AMPA, and kainate subtypes of glutamate receptors are probably all linked to an ion channel. The metabotropic glutamate receptor subtype, however, belongs to the G protein–linked superfamily of receptors. The specific functioning of the various subtypes of glutamate receptors is the focus of intense debate. The actions at NMDA receptors will be emphasized here in our discussions on excitotoxicity.

Just as does the GABA-benzodiazepine receptor complex, the NMDA glutamate–calcium channel complex also has multiple receptors surrounding the ion

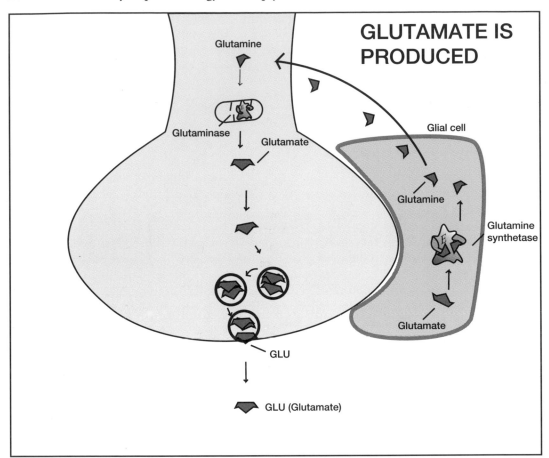

FIGURE 1–21. **Glutamate is produced** (synthesized). Glutamate or glutamic acid (**glu**) is a neurotransmitter that is an amino acid. Its predominant use is not as a neurotransmitter but as an amino acid building block of protein synthesis. When used as a neurotransmitter, it is synthesized from **glutamine**. Glutamine is turned into glutamate by an enzyme present in mitochondria called **glutaminase**. It is then stored in synaptic vesicles for subsequent release during neurotransmission. Glutamine itself can be obtained from glial cells adjacent to neurons. Glial cells have a supportive role to neurons, helping to support them both structurally and metabolically. In the case of glutamate neurons, nearby glia can provide glutamine for neurotransmitter glutamate synthesis. In this case, glutamate from metabolic pools in the glia is converted into glutamate for use as a neurotransmitter. This is accomplished by first converting glutamate into glutamine in the glial cell via the enzyme **glutamine synthetase**. Glutamine is then transported into the neuron for conversion into glutamate for use as a neurotransmitter.

channel, which act in concert as *allosteric modulators* (Fig. 1–24). One modulatory site is for the neurotransmitter *glycine*; another is for *polyamines*, and yet another is for *zinc* (Fig. 1–24). The *magnesium* ion can block the calcium channel at yet another modulatory site, which is presumably inside the ion channel or closely related to it. Another inhibitory modulatory site, located inside the ion

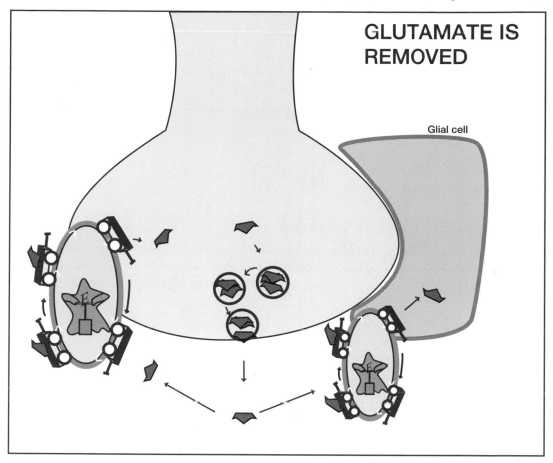

GLUTAMATE IS REMOVED

Glial cell

FIGURE 1–22. **Glutamate removal**. Glutamate's actions are stopped, not by enzymatic breakdown as in other neurotransmitter systems, but by removal by two transport pumps. The first of these pumps is a presynaptic glutamate transporter, which works in the same way as all the other neurotransmitter transporters for monoamine neurotransmitter systems such as dopamine, norepinephrine, and serotonin. The second transport pump, located on nearby glia, removes glutamate from the synapse and terminates its actions there.

channel, is sometimes called the *PCP site* since the psychotomimic agent phencylclidine (PCP) binds to this site (Fig. 1–24). Since PCP induces a psychotic state with some similarities to schizophrenia, it is possible that such psychotic symptoms in schizophrenia may be modulated by dysfunction in the NMDA subtype of glutamate receptor.

Antagonists for any of the various modulatory sites around the NMDA–calcium channel complex would possibly restrict the flow of calcium and close the channel and therefore be candidates for neuroprotective agents. Such antagonists are being developed and tested in various disorders hypothesized to be mediated by an excitotoxic mechanism, such as schizophrenia and Alzheimer's disease.

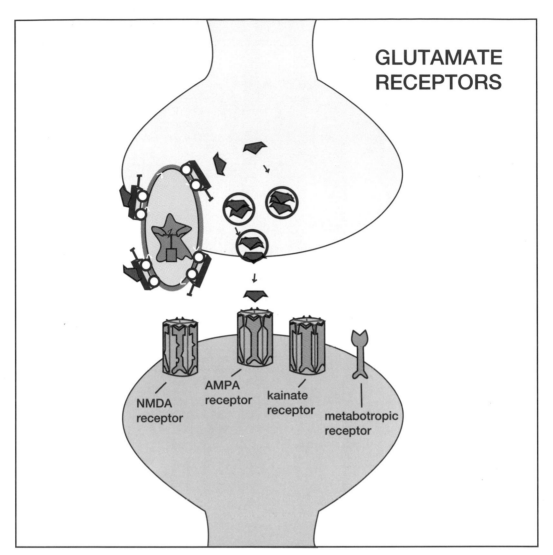

GLUTAMATE
RECEPTORS

NMDA
receptor

AMPA
receptor

kainate
receptor

metabotropic
receptor

FIGURE 1–23. **Glutamate receptors**. There are several types of glutamate receptors, including three that are linked to ion channels: N-methyl-*d*-aspartate (NMDA), alpha-amino-3-hydroxy-5-methyl-4-isoxazolepropionic acid (AMPA), and **kainate**, all named after the agonists that selectively bind to them. Another type of glutamate receptor is the **metabotropic** glutamate receptor, which is a G protein–linked receptor and which may mediate long-lasting electrical signals in the brain by a process called long-term potentiation, which appears to have a key role in memory functions.

FIGURE 1–24. **Five modulatory sites on the N-methyl-*d*-aspartate (NMDA) receptor**. The NMDA glutamate–calcium channel complex has multiple receptors in and around it, which act in concert as **allosteric modulators**. Three of these modulatory sites are located around the NMDA receptor. One of these modulatory sites is for the neurotransmitter **glycine**, another is for **polyamines**, and yet another is for **zinc**. Two of the modulatory sites are located inside or near the ion channel itself. The **magnesium** ion can block the calcium channel at one of these modulatory site, which is presumably inside the ion channel or close to it. The other inhibitory modulatory site, located inside the ion channel, is sometimes called the **PCP site**, since the psychotomimic agent phencylclidine (PCP) binds to this site.

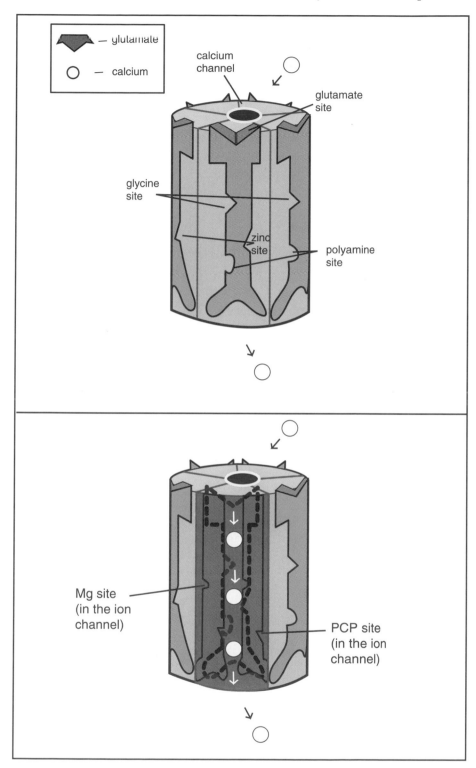

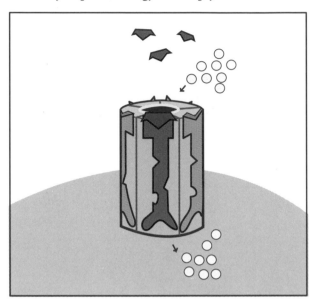

Normal excitatory
neurotransmission

FIGURE 1–25. Shown here is **normal excitatory neurotransmission** at the N-methyl-*d*-aspartate (NMDA) type of glutamate receptor. The NMDA receptor is a **ligand-gated ion channel**. This rapidly transmitting ion channel is an **excitatory** calcium channel. Occupancy of NMDA glutamate receptors by glutamate causes calcium channels to open and the neuron to be excited for neurotransmission.

Excitotoxicity and the glutamate system in neurodegenerative disorders such as schizophrenia. The NMDA subtype of glutamate receptor is thought to mediate normal excitatory neurotransmission (Fig. 1–25) as well as neurodegenerative excitotoxicity in the glutamate excitation spectrum shown in Figure 1–26. Excitotoxicity could mediate the final common pathway of any number of neurological and psychiatric disorders characterized by a neurodegenerative course. The basic idea is that the normal process of excitatory neurotransmission runs amok. Instead of normal excitatory neurotransmission, things get out of hand, and the neuron is literally excited to death (Fig. 1–26). The excitotoxic mechanism is thought to begin with a pathological process which eventually triggers reckless glutamate activity (starting with Fig. 1–27). This could cause dangerous opening of the calcium channel, because if too much calcium enters the cell through open channels, it would poison the cell by activating intracellular enzymes (Fig. 1–28) that form potentially dangerous free radicals (Fig. 1–29). Too many free radicals would eventually overwhelm the cell with toxic actions on cellular membranes and organelles (Fig. 1–30), ultimately killing the cell (Fig. 1–31).

A limited form of excitotoxicity may be useful as a "pruning" mechanism for normal maintenance of the dendritic tree, getting rid of cerebral "dead wood" like a good gardener; however, excitotoxicity to an excess is hypothesized to cause various forms of neurodegeneration, ranging from slow, relentless neurodegenerative conditions such as schizophrenia and Alzheimer's disease to sudden, catastrophic neuronal death such as stroke (Fig. 1–26).

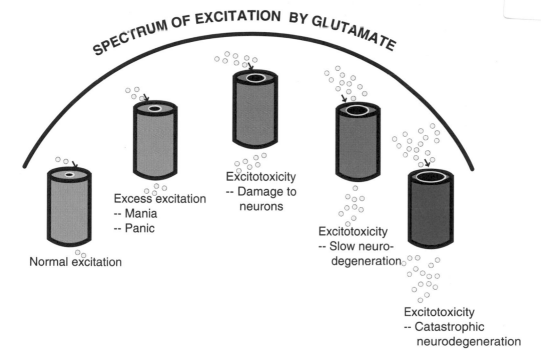

SPECTRUM OF EXCITATION BY GLUTAMATE

Normal excitation

Excess excitation
-- Mania
-- Panic

Excitotoxicity
-- Damage to
neurons

Excitotoxicity
-- Slow neuro-
degeneration

Excitotoxicity
-- Catastrophic
neurodegeneration

FIGURE 1–26. **Neuroprotection, excitotoxicity, and the glutamate system in degenerative disorders**. A major research strategy for the discovery of novel therapeutics in Alzheimer's disease is to target the glutamate system, which might mediate progressive neurodegeneration by an excitotoxic mechanism. Such an excitotoxic mechanism may play a role in various other neurodegenerative diseases such as schizophrenia, Parkinson's disease, Huntington's disease, amyotrophic lateral sclerosis, and even stroke. The **spectrum of excitation by glutamate** ranges from **normal neurotransmission**; to excess neurotransmission, causing pathological symptoms such as **mania** or **panic**; to excitotoxicity, resulting in **minor damage to dendrites**; to **slow progressive excitotoxicity**, resulting in neuronal degeneration such as occurs in Alzheimer's disease; to **sudden and catastrophic excitotoxicity** causing neurodegeneration, as in stroke.

Experimental Therapeutic Approaches

Blocking Neurodegeneration and Apoptosis: Glutamate Antagonists, Free-Radical Scavengers, and Caspase Inhibitors

Various experimental therapeutics based on glutamate, excitotoxicity, and free radicals are being developed. It is possible that glutamate antagonists, especially NMDA antagonists, as well as various antagonists of other allosteric sites at the NMDA receptor, such as the glycine site, may be neuroprotective (Fig. 1–32). Such compounds have been tested in animal models and are in development for human conditions ranging from stroke to schizophrenia to Alzheimer's disease. Some drugs are under development as free-radical scavengers, which have the chemical property of being able to soak up and neutralize toxic free radicals like a chemical sponge and remove them (Fig. 1–33). A weak scavenger that has been tested in Parkinson's disease and tardive dyskinesia is vitamin E. A more powerful set of agents are the

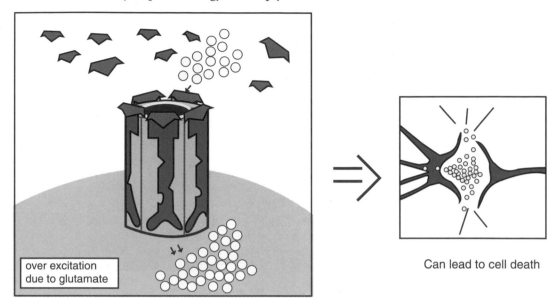

over excitation
due to glutamate

Can lead to cell death

FIGURE 1–27. **Cellular events occurring during excitotoxicity (part 1).** Excitotoxicity is a major current hypothesis for explaining a neuropathological mechanism that could mediate the final common pathway of any number of neurological and psychiatric disorders characterized by a neurodegenerative course. The basic idea is that the normal process of excitatory neurotransmission runs amok, and instead of normal excitatory neurotransmission, things get out of hand and the neuron is literally excited to death. The excitotoxic mechanism is thought to begin with a pathological process that triggers excessive glutamate activity. This causes excessive opening of the calcium channel, shown here, beginning the process of poisoning of the cell by allowing too much calcium to enter it.

lazaroids (so named because of their putative actions of raising degenerating neurons, like Lazarus, from the dead). Another therapeutic approach has to do with blocking the enzyme system that may be necessary for apoptosis to occur, namely the caspase enzymes.

Presymptomatic Treatment

One idea that is gaining interest and generating debate is the possibility of intervening early in the course of schizophrenia by treating with atypical antipsychotic agents during the prodromal phase prior to the onset of active psychotic symptoms (see Fig. 1–20, stage II). This strategy is causing debate, and even controversy, for there is no assurance that early intervention will lead to improved outcomes, especially since diagnosis of schizophrenia is not very accurate at this point in the illness. Nevertheless, since it is theoretically possible that psychosis itself could be damaging to the brain as a result of excitotoxic neuronal destruction during acute psychosis, there is the provocative possibility that one might be able to abort the illness and modify its natural history by early intervention. It seems obvious that psychosis is not good for the brain, as exemplified by data from studies showing that patients who are ill for a shorter time prior to initiating treatment with antipsychotic drugs are more likely to respond to them than are those with longer duration

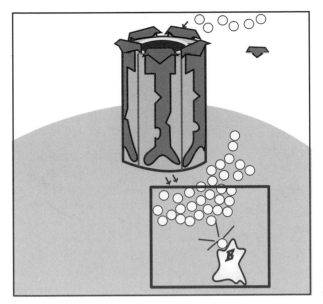

Excess calcium
activates enzyme

FIGURE 1–28. **Cellular events occurring during excitotoxicity (part 2).** The internal milieu of a neuron is very sensitive to calcium, as a small increase in calcium concentration will alter all sorts of enzyme activity, as well as neuronal membrane excitability. If calcium levels rise too much, they will begin to activate enzymes that can be dangerous for the cell owing to their ability to trigger a destructive chemical cascade.

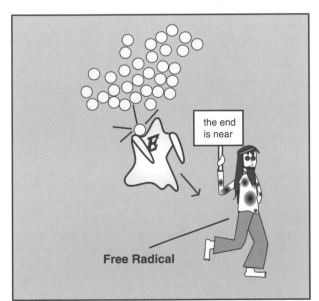

the end
is near

Enzyme produces
free radical

Free Radical

FIGURE 1–29. **Cellular events occurring during excitotoxicity (part 3).** Once excessive glutamate causes too much calcium to enter the neuron and calcium **activates dangerous enzymes, these enzymes go on to produce troublesome free radicals.** Free radicals are chemicals that are capable of destroying other cellular components, such as organelles and membranes, by destructive chemical reactions.

31

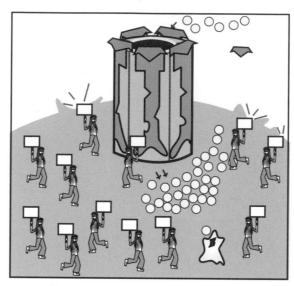

Free radicals begin destroying the cell

FIGURE 1–30. **Cellular events occurring during excitotoxicity (part 4).** As the calcium accumulates in the cell, and the enzymes produce more and more free radicals, they begin to indiscriminately destroy parts of the cell, especially its neuronal and nuclear membranes and critical organelles such as energy-producing mitochondria.

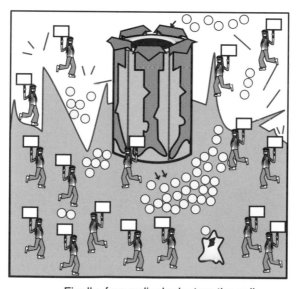

Finally, free radicals destroy the cell

FIGURE 1–31. **Cellular events occurring during excitotoxicity (part 5).** Eventually, the damage is so great that the free radicals essentially destroy the whole neuron.

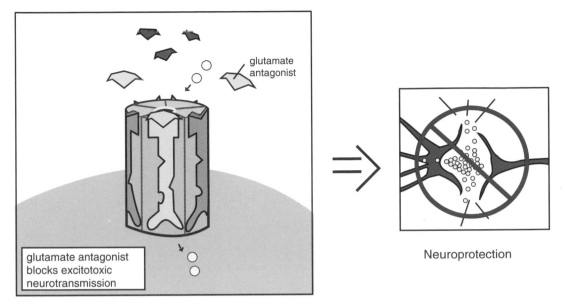

FIGURE 1–32. Glutamate antagonists. **Antagonists of glutamate** at the NMDA agonist site can block excitotoxic neurotransmission and exert neuroprotective actions. Such drugs stop excessive calcium entry and its consequences. These agents are in experimental testing for various neurodegenerative disorders and stroke.

of symptoms before treatment is begun. This suggests that an active phase of schizophrenia may reflect a morbid process that begins as early as the prodromal/presymptomatic stage, and which if allowed to persist, can impair the patient's ability to respond to treatment when finally instituted. Some investigators are even extending these ideas to interventions aimed at relatively asymptomatic first-degree relatives of persons with many schizophrenic patients in the family. Whether it will ever be possible to modify or abort the course of schizophrenia is an exciting if perplexing methodological issue for future research.

Combined Neurodevelopmental/Neurodegenerative Hypothesis

It may be difficult to conceive of a purely neurodevelopmental process that would be completed early in life, that would be entirely asymptomatic until the disease process begins, and that would generate a downhill course and waxing and waning symptomatology. Thus, schizophrenia may be a neurodegenerative process superimposed on a neurodevelopmental abnormality (Fig. 1–34). Candidate neurons for the site of neurodegeneration include dopamine projections to the cortex and glutamate projections back from the cortex to subcortical structures. It is even possible that excitotoxicity occurs in these structures when positive symptoms are produced during psychotic relapses.

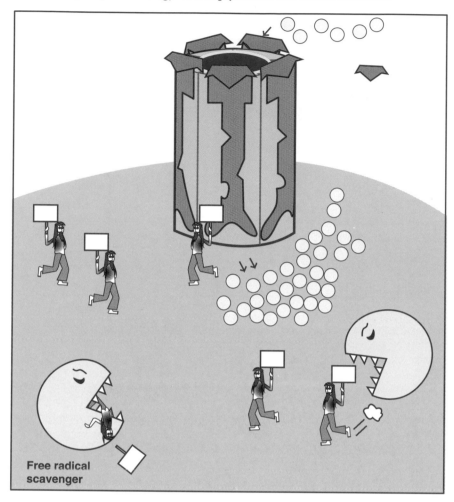

FIGURE 1–33. **Free radicals** are generated in the neurodegenerative process of excitotoxicity. A drug acting as a **free-radical scavenger**, which acts as a chemical sponge by soaking up toxic free radicals and removing them, would be neuroprotective. Vitamin E is a weak scavenger. Other free-radical scavengers, such as the lazaroids (so named because of their putative properties of raising degenerating neurons, like Lazarus, from the dead) are also being tested.

Summary

This chapter has provided a clinical description of psychosis, with special emphasis on the psychotic illness schizophrenia. We have explained the dopamine hypothesis of schizophrenia, which is the major hypothesis for explaining the mechanism for the positive symptoms of psychosis (delusions and hallucinations).

The four major dopamine pathways in the brain have been described. The mesolimbic dopamine system, which may mediate the positive symptoms of psychosis; the mesocortical system, which may mediate the negative symptoms and cognitive symptoms of psychosis; the nigrostriatal system, which mediates extrapyramidal

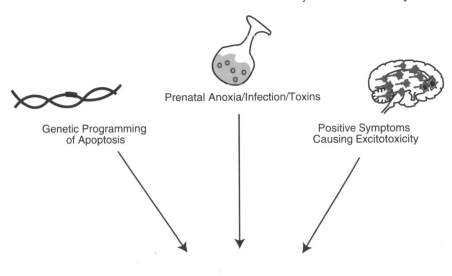

Genetic Programming
of Apoptosis

Prenatal Anoxia/Infection/Toxins

Positive Symptoms
Causing Excitotoxicity

Dead Neuron or Loss of Dendrites

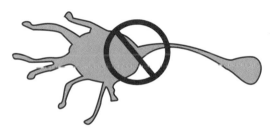

FIGURE 1–34. **Neurodegenerative causes of schizophrenia** may lead to a final common pathway either of neuronal death or possibly of destruction of synapses and the axons and dendrites of such synapses. The causes can range from predetermined genetic programming of neuronal or synaptic destruction; to fetal insults such as anoxia, infection, toxins, or maternal starvation; to perhaps a destructive effect of the positive symptoms themselves on synapses and neurons via glutamate-mediated excitotoxicity.

movement disorders such as Parkinson's disease and tardive dyskinesia; and the tuberoinfundibular system, which controls plasma prolactin levels.

We have also developed the major neurodevelopmental and neurodegenerative hypotheses for schizophrenia and have explained glutamate neurotransmission and the phenomenon of excitotoxicity.

ANTIPSYCHOTIC AGENTS

This chapter will explore the various drug treatments for psychotic disorders, with special emphasis on schizophrenia. Such treatments include not only conventional antipsychotic drugs but also the newer atypical antipsychotic drugs, which are rapidly replacing the older conventional agents. We will also take a look into the future at the drugs under development for psychosis, especially schizophrenia.

The specifics of antipsychotic drug treatments will differ, of course, depending on the psychotic disorder (i.e., schizophrenia or other), as well as on how the patient has responded to treatments in the past. Economic considerations are unfortunately also a factor, as the newer drugs are quite expensive; fortunately, they may reduce the overall cost of treatment. Also, antipsychotic treatments can vary, notably in terms of how individual patients respond to specific antipsychotic drugs, doses, durations of treatment, and combinations with additional psychotropic medications. The reader is referred to standard reference manuals and textbooks for practical prescribing information, such as drug doses, because this chapter will emphasize basic pharmacologic concepts of mechanisms of action and not practical issues such as to how to prescribe these drugs. The pharmacological concepts developed here should, however, help the reader understand the rationale for how to use antipsychotic agents based on their interactions with different neurotransmitter systems in the central nervous system. Such interactions can often explain both the therapeutic actions and side effects of antipsychotic medications and are thus very helpful background information for prescribers.

Conventional Antipsychotic Drugs

The earliest effective treatments for schizophrenia and other psychotic illnesses arose from serendipitous clinical observations rather than from scientific knowledge of the neurobiological basis of psychosis or the mechanism of action of effective antipsychotic agents. Thus, the first antipsychotic drugs were discovered by accident in the 1950s when a putative antihistamine (chlorpromazine) was serendipitously observed to have antipsychotic effects when tested in schizophrenic patients. Chlorpromazine indeed has antihistaminic activity, but its therapeutic actions in schizophrenia are not mediated by this property. Once chlorpromazine was observed to be an effective antipsychotic agent, it was tested experimentally to uncover its mechanism of antipsychotic action.

Early in the testing process, chlorpromazine and other antipsychotic agents were all found to cause *neurolepsis*, known as an extreme slowness or absence of motor movements as well as behavioral indifference in experimental animals. The original antipsychotics were first discovered largely by their ability to produce this effect in experimental animals and are thus sometimes called neuroleptics. A human counterpart of neurolepsis is also caused by these original (i.e., conventional) antipsychotic drugs and is characterized by psychomotor slowing, emotional quieting, and affective indifference.

Blockade of Dopamine 2 Receptors as the Mechanism of Action of Conventional Antipsychotics

By the late 1960s and 1970s it was widely recognized that the key pharmacologic property of all neuroleptics with antipsychotic properties was their ability to block dopamine 2 receptors (Fig. 2–1). This action has proved to be responsible not only for the antipsychotic efficacy of conventional antipsychotic drugs but also for most of their undesirable side effects, including neurolepsis.

The therapeutic actions of conventional antipsychotic drugs are due to blockade of D2 receptors specifically in the mesolimbic dopamine pathway (Fig. 2–2). This has the effect of reducing the hyperactivity in this pathway that is postulated to cause the positive symptoms of psychosis, as discussed in Chapter 1 (see Figs. 1–8 and 1–9). All conventional antipsychotics reduced positive psychotic symptoms about equally in schizophrenic patients who were studied in large multicenter trials. That is not to say that one individual patient might not occasionally respond better to one conventional antipsychotic agent than to another, but there is no consistent difference in antipsychotic efficacy among the conventional antipsychotic agents. A list of many conventional antipsychotic drugs is given in Table 2–1.

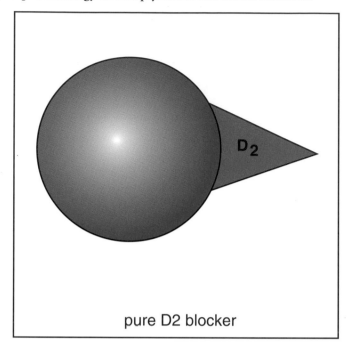

FIGURE 2–1. This icon represents the notion of a single pharmacologic action, namely *dopamine 2 (D2) receptor antagonism*. Although actual drugs have multiple pharmacologic action, this single action idea will be applied conceptually in several of the following figures.

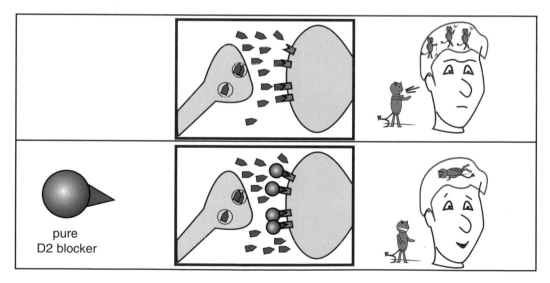

FIGURE 2–2. The *dopamine receptor antagonist hypothesis* of antipsychotic drug action for *positive symptoms* of psychosis in the *mesolimbic* dopamine pathway is shown here. Blockade of postsynaptic dopamine 2 receptors by a dopamine 2 antagonist acting in the mesolimbic dopamine pathway is hypothesized to mediate the antipsychotic efficacy of the antipsychotic drugs and their ability to diminish or block positive symptoms.

Table 2–1. *Conventional antipsychotic agents used to treat psychosis and schizophrenia in the United States*

Generic Name	Trade Name
Acetophenazine	Tindal
Carphenazine	Proketazine
Chlorpromazine	Thorazine
Chlorprothixene	Taractan
Clozapine	Clozaril
Fluphenazine	Prolixin; Permitil
Haloperidol	Haldol
Loxapine	Loxitane
Mesoridazine	Serentil
Molindone	Moban; Lidone
Perphenazine	Trilafon
Pimozide	Orap[a]
Piperacetazine	Quide
Prochlorperazine	Compazine[b]
Thioridazine	Mellaril
Thiothixene	Navane
Trifluoperazine	Stelazine
Triflupromazine	Vesprin

[a]Approved in the United States for Tourette syndrome.
[b]Approved in the United States for nausea and vomiting as well as psychosis.

Unfortunately, it is not possible to block just these D2 receptors in the mesolimbic dopamine (DA) pathway with conventional antipsychotics because these drugs are delivered throughout the entire brain after oral ingestion. Thus, conventional antipsychotics will seek out every D2 receptor throughout the brain and block them all (see Fig. 1–7). This leads to a high "cost of doing business" in order to get the mesolimbic D2 receptors blocked.

Specifically, the D2 receptors will also be blocked in the mesocortical DA pathway (Fig. 2–3), where DA may already be deficient in schizophrenia (see Figs. 1–10 and 1–11). When this happens, it can cause or worsen negative and cognitive symptoms. This is sometimes called the *neuroleptic-induced deficit syndrome* because it looks so much like the negative symptoms produced by schizophrenia itself and is reminiscent of neurolepsis in animals.

When D2 receptors are blocked in the nigrostriatal DA pathway, it produces disorders of movement that can appear very much like those in Parkinson's disease; this is why these movements are sometimes called drug-induced parkinsonism (Fig. 2–4). Since the nigrostriatal pathway is part of the extrapyramidal nervous system, these motor side effects associated with blocking of D2 receptors in this part of the brain are sometimes also called extrapyramidal symptoms, or EPS.

Mesocortical pathway

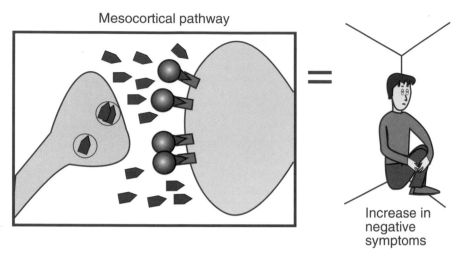

Increase in negative symptoms

FIGURE 2–3. When **postsynaptic dopamine 2 receptors** are blocked by dopamine 2 antagonist acting in the **mesocortical** dopamine pathway, this can cause emotional blunting and cognitive problems that mimic the **negative symptoms** of schizophrenia. Sometimes these cognitive side effects of antipsychotics are called the "neuroleptic induced deficit syndrome." If a patient already has these symptoms before treatment, medication with drugs that block these receptors can make their negative symptoms worse.

Nigrostriatal pathway

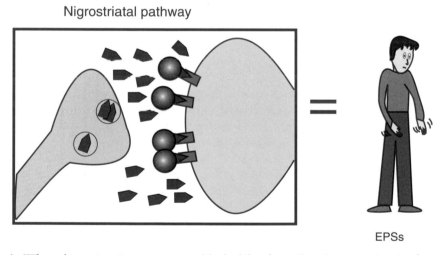

EPSs

FIGURE 2–4. When dopamine 2 receptors are blocked by dopamine 2 antagonists in the postsynaptic projections of the *nigrostriatal* pathway, it produces disorders of movement, which can appear very much like those in Parkinson's disease. That is why these movements are sometimes called drug-induced parkinsonism. Since the nigrostriatal pathway projects to the basal ganglia, a part of the so-called extrapyramidal nervous system, side effects associated with blockade of dopamine 2 receptors there are sometimes also called extrapyramidal symptoms (EPS).

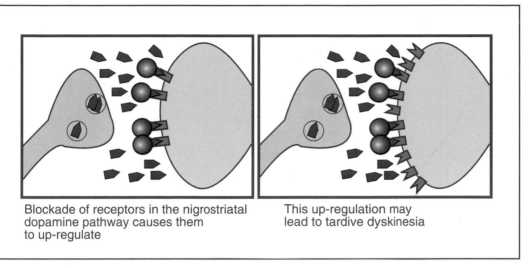

Blockade of receptors in the nigrostriatal dopamine pathway causes them to up-regulate

This up-regulation may lead to tardive dyskinesia

FIGURE 2–5. **Long-term** blockade of dopamine 2 receptors by dopamine 2 antagonists in the **nigrostriatal** dopamine pathway may cause these receptors to up-regulate. A clinical consequence of this may be the hyperkinetic movement disorder known as **tardive dyskinesia**. This up-regulation may be the consequence of the neuron's futile attempt to overcome drug-induced blockade of its dopamine receptors.

Worse yet, if these D2 receptors in the nigrostriatal DA pathway are blocked chronically (Fig. 2–5), they can produce a hyperkinetic movement disorder known as *tardive dyskinesia*. This movement disorder causes facial and tongue movements such as constant chewing, tongue protrusions, and facial grimacing, as well as limb movements, which can be quick, jerky or choreiform (dancing). Tardive dyskinesia is thus caused by long-term administration of conventional antipsychotics and is thought to be mediated by changes, sometimes irreversible, in the D2 receptors of the nigrostriatal DA pathway. Specifically, these receptors are hypothesized to become supersensitive or to up-regulate (i.e., increase in number), perhaps in a futile attempt to overcome drug-induced blockade of these receptors (Fig. 2–5).

About 5% of patients maintained on conventional antipsychotics will develop tardive dyskinesia every year (i.e., 20% by 4 years), which is not a very encouraging prospect for a lifelong illness starting in the early twenties. If the D2 receptor blockade is removed early enough, tardive dyskinesia may reverse. This reversal is theoretically due to resetting of these receptors by an appropriate decrease in the number or sensitivity of D2 receptors in the nigrostriatal pathway once the antipsychotic drugs that had been blocking these receptors are removed. However, after long-term treatment, the D2 receptors apparently cannot or do not reset back to normal, even when conventional antipsychotic drugs are discontinued. This leads to irreversible tardive dyskinesia, which continues whether conventional antipsychotic drugs are administered or not.

Dopamine 2 receptors in the fourth DA pathway, namely the tuberoinfundibular DA pathway, are also blocked by conventional antipsychotics, and this causes plasma prolactin concentrations to rise, a condition called *hyperprolactinemia* (Fig. 2–6). This is associated with conditions called galactorrhea (breast secretions) and amenorrhea

Tuberoinfundibular pathway

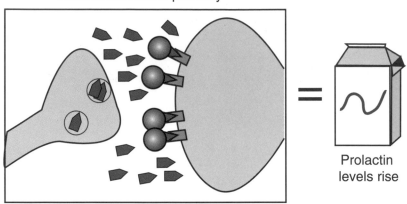

Prolactin
levels rise

FIGURE 2–6. The **tuberoinfundibular** dopamine pathway controls **prolactin** secretion. When dopamine 2 receptors in this pathway are blocked by dopamine 2 antagonists, prolactin levels rise, sometimes so much so that women may begin lactating inappropriately, a condition known as galactorrhea.

(irregular menstrual periods). Hyperprolactinemia may thus interfere with fertility, especially in women. Hyperprolactinemia might lead to more rapid demineralization of bones in postmenopausal women who are not receiving estrogen replacement therapy. Other possible problems associated with elevated prolactin levels include sexual dysfunction and weight gain, although the role of prolactin in causing such problems is not clear.

The Dilemma of Blocking D2 Dopamine Receptors in All Four Dopamine Pathways

It should now be obvious that the use of conventional antipsychotic drugs presents a powerful dilemma. That is, there is no doubt that conventional antipsychotic medications have dramatic therapeutic actions on positive symptoms of psychosis by blocking hyperactive dopamine neurons in the mesolimbic dopamine pathway. However, there are four dopamine pathways in the brain, and it appears that blocking dopamine receptors in only one of them is useful, whereas blocking dopamine receptors in the remaining three pathways may be harmful.

Specifically, while delusions and hallucinations are reduced when mesolimbic D2 receptors are blocked, negative and cognitive symptoms of psychosis may be worsened when mesocortical D2 receptors are blocked; EPS and tardive dyskinesia may be produced when nigrostriatal D2 receptors are blocked; and hyperprolactinemia and its complications may be produced when tuberoinfundibular D2 receptors are blocked. The pharmacologic quandary here is: What should one do if one wishes to decrease dopamine in the mesolimbic dopamine pathway in order to treat positive psychotic symptoms, which are theoretically mediated by hyperactive mesolimbic dopamine neurons, and yet simultaneously increase dopamine in the mesocortical dopamine pathway to treat negative and cognitive symptoms, while leaving dopaminergic tone unchanged in both the nigrostriatal and tuberoin-fundibular dopamine pathways to avoid side effects?

This dilemma may have been solved in part by the atypical antipsychotic drugs described in the following section and is one of the reasons why the atypical antipsychotic agents are rapidly replacing the conventional ones in the treatment of schizophrenia and other psychotic disorders throughout the world.

Risks and Benefits of Long-Term Treatment with Conventional Antipsychotics

Although the conventional antipsychotics reduce positive psychotic symptoms in most patients after several weeks of treatment, discontinuing these drugs causes relapse of psychosis in schizophrenic patients at the rate of approximately 10% per month, so that 50% or more have relapsed by 6 months after medication is discontinued. Despite this powerful incentive for patients to continue long-term treatment with conventional antipsychotics to prevent relapse, the unfortunate fact that all four dopamine pathways are blocked by these drugs means that the trade-off for many patients is that the benefits of long-term treatment are not considered worth the problems they cause. This leads many patients to discontinue treatment, become noncompliant, and relapse, with a "revolving door" lifestyle in and out of the hospital. Patients too commonly select the risk of relapse over subjectively unacceptable side effects of the conventional antipsychotics. Especially unacceptable to patients are motor restlessness and EPS such as akathisia, rigidity, and tremor, as well as cognitive blunting and social withdrawal, anhedonia, and apathy. There is even the possibility of a rare but potentially fatal complication called the *neuroleptic malignant syndrome*, which is associated with extreme muscular rigidity, high fever, coma, and even death. Fortunately, the burden of side effects with treatment by atypical antipsychotics appears to be much less than that with conventional antipsychotics and can lead to better compliance and long-term outcomes, as discussed in the next section on atypical antipsychotic drugs.

Muscarinic Cholinergic Blocking Properties of Conventional Antipsychotics

In addition to blocking D2 receptors in all four dopamine pathways, conventional antipsychotics have other important pharmacologic properties (Fig. 2–7). One particularly important pharmacologic action of some conventional antipsychotics is their ability to block muscarinic cholinergic receptors. This can cause undesirable side effects, such as dry mouth, blurred vision, constipation, and cognitive blunting (Fig. 2–8). Differing degrees of muscarinic cholinergic blockade may also explain why some conventional antipsychotics have a greater propensity to produce extrapyramidal side effects than others. That is, those conventional antipsychotics that cause more EPS are the agents that have only weak anticholinergic properties, whereas those conventional antipsychotics that cause fewer EPS are the agents that have stronger anticholinergic properties.

How does muscarinic cholinergic receptor blockade reduce the EPS caused by dopamine D2 receptor blockade in the nigrostriatal pathway? The reason seems to be that dopamine and acetylcholine have a reciprocal relationship in the nigrostriatal

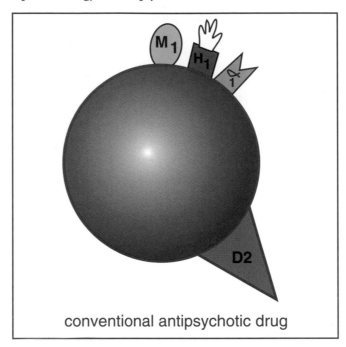

conventional antipsychotic drug

FIGURE 2–7. This figure represents an icon of a **conventional antipsychotic drug**. Such drugs generally have at least four actions: blockade of dopamine 2 receptors (D2); blockade of muscarinic-cholinergic receptors (M1); blockade of alpha 1 adrenergic receptors (alpha 1); and blockade of histamine receptors (antihistaminic actions; [H1]).

pathway (see Figs. 2–9 to 2–11). Dopamine neurons in the nigrostriatal dopamine pathway make postsynaptic connections with cholinergic neurons (Fig. 2–9). Dopamine normally inhibits acetylcholine release from postsynaptic nigrostriatal cholinergic neurons, thus suppressing acetylcholine activity there (Fig. 2–9). If dopamine can no longer suppress acetylcholine release because dopamine receptors are being blocked by a conventional antipsychotic drug, then acetylcholine becomes overly active (Fig. 2–10).

One way to compensate for this overactivity of acetylcholine is to block it with an anticholinergic agent (Fig. 2–11). Thus, drugs with anticholinergic actions will diminish the excess acetylcholine activity caused by removal of dopamine inhibition when dopamine receptors are blocked (Fig. 2–11). If anticholinergic properties are present in the same drug with D2 blocking properties, they will tend to mitigate the effects of D2 blockade in the nigrostriatal dopamine pathway. Thus, conventional antipsychotics with potent anticholinergic properties have lower EPS than conventional antipsychotics with weak anticholinergic properties. Furthermore, the effects of D2 blockade in the nigrostriatal system can be mitigated by coadministering an agent with anticholinergic properties. This has led to the common strategy of giving anticholinergic agents along with conventional antipsychotics in order to reduce EPS. Unfortunately, this concomitant use of anticholinergic agents does not lessen the ability of the conventional antipsychotics to cause tardive dyskinesia. It also causes the well-known side effects associated with anticholinergic

M1 INSERTED

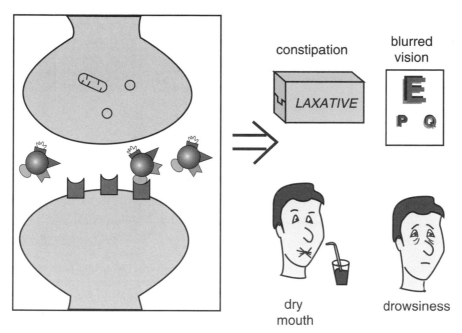

FIGURE 2–8. *Side effects of the conventional antipsychotics* (part 1). In this diagram, the icon of a conventional antipsychotic drug is shown with its M1 anticholinergic-antimuscarinic portion inserted into acetylcholine receptors, causing the side effects of constipation, blurred vision, dry mouth, and drowsiness.

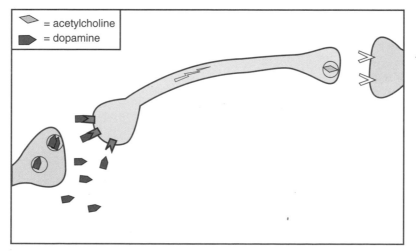

FIGURE 2–9. **Dopamine and acetylcholine** have a reciprocal relationship in the nigrostriatal dopamine pathway. Dopamine neurons here make postsynaptic connections with cholinergic neurons. Normally, **dopamine suppresses acetylcholine** activity.

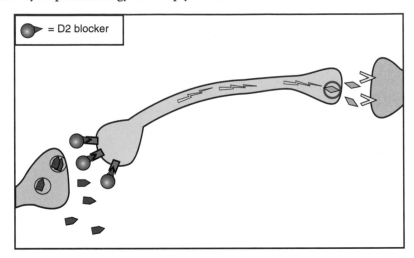

FIGURE 2–10. This figure shows what happens to acetylcholine activity when **dopamine receptors are blocked**. As dopamine normally suppresses acetylcholine activity, removal of dopamine inhibition causes an **increase in acetylcholine** activity. Thus, if dopamine receptors are blocked, acetylcholine becomes overly active. This is associated with the production of extrapyramidal symptoms (EPS). The pharmacological mechanism of EPS therefore seems to be a relative dopamine deficiency and an acetylcholine excess.

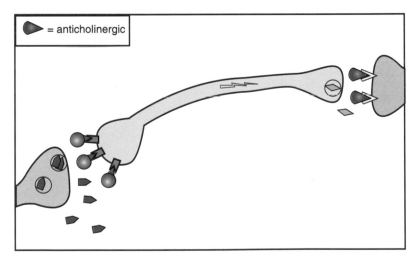

FIGURE 2–11. One **compensation** for the overactivity of acetylcholine that occurs when dopamine receptors are blocked is to block the acetylcholine receptors with an **anticholinergic agent**. Thus, anticholinergics overcome excess acetylcholine activity caused by removal of dopamine inhibition when dopamine receptors are blocked by conventional antipsychotics. This also means that extrapyramidal symptoms (EPS) are reduced.

H1 INSERTED

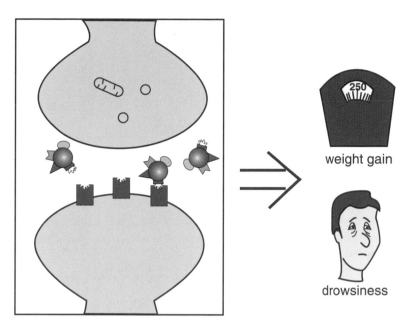

FIGURE 2–12. *Side effects of conventional antipsychotics*, part 2. In this diagram, the icon of a conventional antipsychotic drug is shown with its H1 (antihistamine) portion inserted into histamine receptors, causing the side effects of weight gain and drowsiness.

agents, such as dry mouth, blurred vision, constipation, urinary retention, and cognitive dysfunction.

Other Pharmacologic Properties of Conventional Antipsychotic Drugs

Still other pharmacologic actions are associated with the conventional antipsychotic drugs. These include generally undesired activity at alpha 1 adrenergic receptors as well as at histamine 1 receptors, as already discussed (Fig. 2–7). Thus, conventional antipsychotic drugs have activities at three of the same neurotransmitter receptors that mediate the well characterized side effects of the tricyclic antidepressants. That is, these drugs have antihistaminic properties (causing weight gain and drowsiness) (Fig. 2–12), alpha 1 adrenergic blocking properties (causing cardiovascular side effects such as orthostatic hypotension and drowsiness) (Fig. 2–13), and muscarinic cholinergic blocking properties (causing dry mouth, blurred vision, constipation, urinary retention, and cognitive dysfunction) (Fig. 2–8). Conventional antipsychotic agents differ in terms of their ability to block the various receptors represented in Figure 2–7. For example, the popular conventional antipsychotic haloperidol (Figs. 2–14 and 2–15) has relatively little anticholinergic or antihistaminic binding activity (Fig. 2–15). Because of this, conventional antipsychotics may differ somewhat in their side effect profiles, even if they do not differ overall in their therapeutic profiles. That is, some conventional antipsychotics are more sedating than others; some have more ability to cause cardiovascular side effects than others; and some are more potent than others.

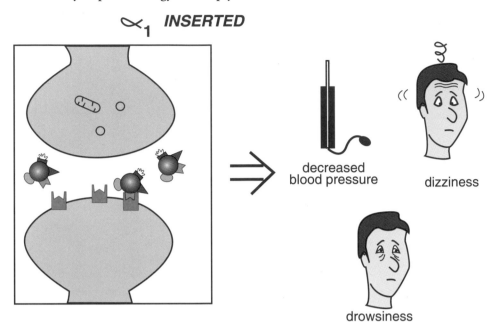

FIGURE 2–13. *Side effects of conventional antipsychotics*, part 3. In this diagram, the icon of a conventional antipsychotic drug is shown with its alpha 1 (alpha 1 antagonist) portion inserted into alpha 1 adrenergic receptors, causing the side effects of dizziness, decreased blood pressure, and drowsiness.

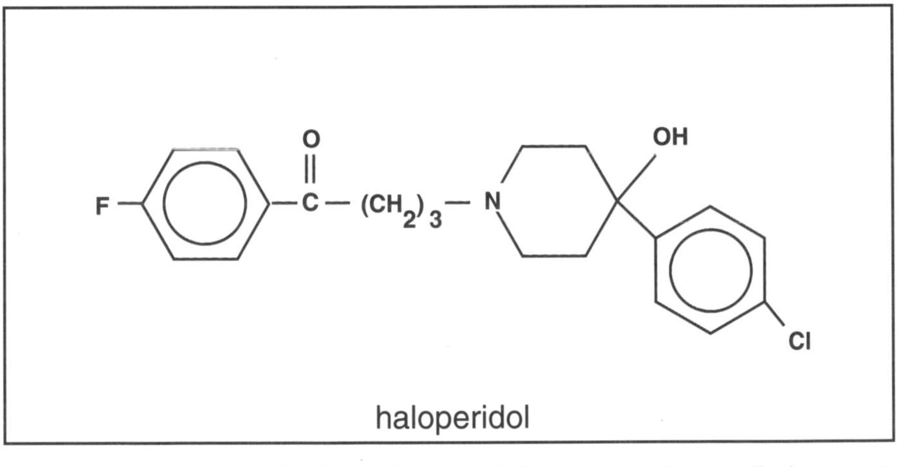

FIGURE 2–14. Structural **formula** of **haloperidol**, one of the most widely prescribed conventional antipsychotic drugs during the height of the conventional antipsychotic era, prior to the mid 1990s.

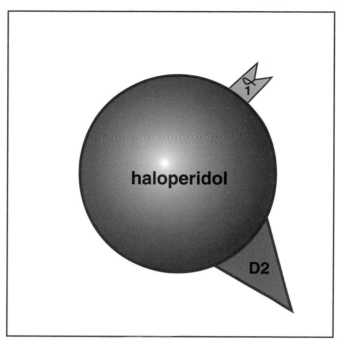

FIGURE 2–15. **Haloperidol** pharmacological icon. Haloperidol is different from many of the other conventional antipsychotic drugs in that it is more potent; it also lacks potent antimuscarinic and antihistaminic binding activities. Otherwise, its clinical profile is highly conventional.

Atypical Antipsychotic Drugs: Serotonin-Dopamine Antagonism and What Several Antipsychotic Drugs Have in Common

What is an atypical antipsychotic? From a pharmacological perspective, the atypical antipsychotics as a class may be defined in part as serotonin-dopamine antagonists (SDAs) (Fig. 2–16). Several other distinguishing pharmacological characteristics will be discussed in the following section. In this section, we will first discuss how the atypical antipsychotics all derive some of their "atypical" clinical properties from exploiting the different ways that serotonin and dopamine interact within the four key dopamine pathways in the brain. Thus, it is very important to understand serotonin-dopamine interactions in each of the four dopamine pathways.

From a clinical perspective, an atypical antipsychotic, however, is defined in part by the clinical properties that distinguish such drugs from conventional antipsychotics, namely, low extrapyramidal symptoms and efficacy for negative symptoms. By understanding the difference between blocking dopamine D2 receptors alone with a conventional antipsychotic versus blocking serotonin 2A receptors and D2 receptors simultaneously with an atypical antipsychotic in the various dopamine pathways (described below), it should be clear why the atypical antipsychotics have several distinct and atypical clinical properties in common. In this section, we will discuss those features shared by the atypical antipsychotics. Later, we will show that atypical antipsychotics also have features that distinguish one from another. Both the overlapping and the distinguishing features are based on pharmacological mechanisms

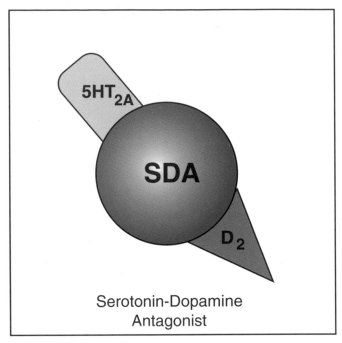

FIGURE 2–16. **Serotonin-dopamine antagonist** (SDA) icon. This icon represents the dual pharmacologic actions that define SDAs, namely blockade of serotonin 2A (5HT2A) receptors, as well as blockade of dopamine 2 (D2) receptors.

and clinical observations. Here we will start with the rules (i.e., similarities among the five atypical antipsychotics clozapine, risperidone, olanzapine, quetiapine, and ziprasidone) before discussing the exceptions (i.e., differences among them). Currently, these are the five drugs in psychiatric practice throughout the world that are considered to be atypical antipsychotics by the following three pharmacologic and clinical criteria: (1) atypical antipsychotics have serotonin 2A–dopamine 2 antagonist pharmacological properties, whereas conventional antipsychotics are only dopamine 2 antagonists; (2) atypical antipsychotics cause fewer EPS than conventional antipsychotics; and (3) atypical antipsychotics improve positive symptoms as well as do conventional antipsychotics. Some may argue that zotepine should be included in this group, as should sertindole, recently withdrawn from marketing with the possibility of returning in the future. These are included in the section on potential new drugs of the future.

Serotonin-Dopamine Antagonism and Serotonergic Control of Dopamine Release in the Four Key Dopamine Pathways

Serotonin has important influences on dopamine, but that influence is quite different in each of the four dopamine pathways. Understanding the differential serotonergic control of dopamine release in each of these four pathways is critical to understanding the differential actions of antipsychotic drugs that block only dopamine 2 receptors (i.e., the conventional antipsychotics) versus antipsychotic

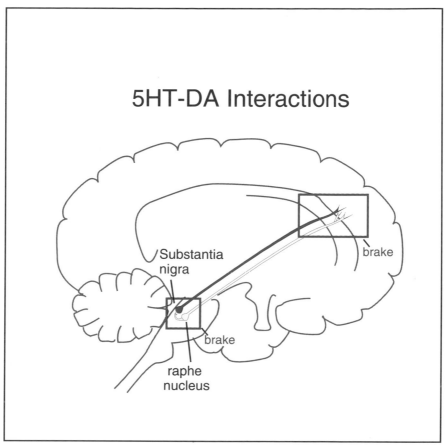

5HT-DA Interactions

Substantia
nigra

brake

brake

raphe
nucleus

FIGURE 2–17. Serotonin-dopamine interactions in the **nigrostriatal** dopamine pathway. **Serotonin inhibits dopamine release**, both at the level of dopamine cell bodies in the brainstem substantia nigra and at the level of the axon terminals in the basal ganglia–neostriatum (see also Figs. 2–18 through 2–20). In both cases, the release of serotonin acts as a **"brake"** on dopamine release.

drugs that block both serotonin 2A and dopamine 2 receptors (i.e., the atypical antipsychotics). That is, serotonin inhibits dopamine release from dopaminergic axon terminals in the various dopamine pathways, but the degree of control differs from one dopamine pathway to another.

Serotonin-Dopamine Interactions in the Nigrostriatal Pathway

Serotonin inhibits dopamine release, both at the level of dopamine cell bodies and at the level of dopaminergic axon terminals (Fig. 2–17). Serotonin neurons from the brainstem raphe innervate the dopamine cell bodies in the substantia nigra and also project to the basal ganglia, where serotonin axon terminals are in close proximity to dopamine axon terminals (Figs. 2–17 to 2–20). In both areas, serotonin interacts with postsynaptic serotonin 2A receptors on the dopamine neuron, and this inhibits dopamine release. Thus, in the nigrostriatal dopamine pathway, serotonin exerts powerful control over dopamine release because it occurs at

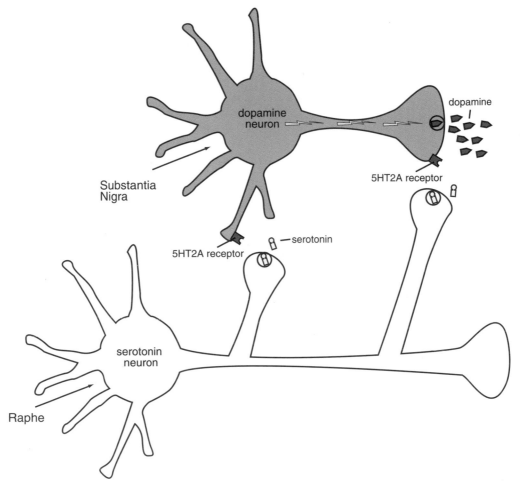

FIGURE 2–18. *Serotonin regulation of dopamine release from nigrostriatal dopamine neurons*, part 1. Here, dopamine is being freely released from its axon terminal in the striatum because there is no serotonin causing any inhibition of dopamine release.

two levels. At the level of serotonergic innervation of the substantia nigra, axon terminals arriving from the raphe synapse on cell bodies and dendrites of dopaminergic cells (Figs. 2–18 to 2–20). At the level of the axon terminals, however, serotonergic interaction with dopamine neurons may be via axoaxonal synapses or via volume (nonsynaptic) neurotransmission from serotonin that diffuses to dopamine axon terminals from nearby serotonin axon terminals but without a synapse (Figs. 2–18 to 2–20). In both cases, however, serotonin interacts via serotonin 2A receptors on the dopamine neuron, which inhibit dopamine release. A close-up of the action of serotonin's inhibitory actions on dopamine release from nigrostriatal dopamine axon terminals is shown in Figs. 2–21 and 2–22.

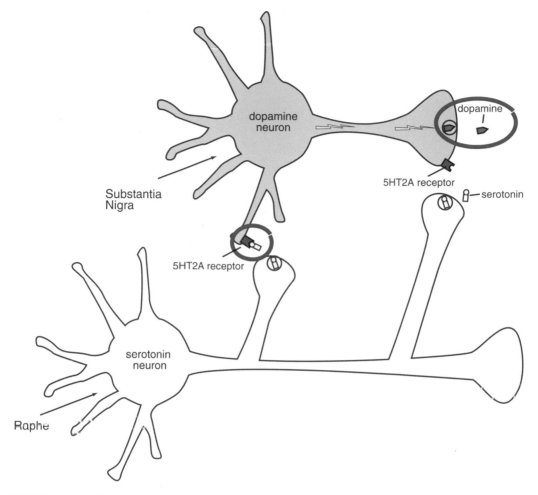

FIGURE 2–19. *Serotonin regulation of dopamine release from nigrostriatal dopamine neurons*, part 2. Now, serotonin is being released from a synaptic connection projecting from the raphe to the substantia nigra and terminating on a postsynaptic serotonin 2A (5HT2A) receptor (*bottom red circle*). Because of this, dopamine release from its axonal terminal is now inhibited (*top red circle*).

The Nigrostriatal Pathway and the Pharmacology of Low Extrapyramidal Symptoms

Serotonin 2A antagonism fortunately reverses dopamine 2 antagonism in the nigrostriatal dopamine pathway. Since stimulating 5HT2A receptors inhibits dopamine release (e.g., Fig. 2–22), it would make sense that the opposite would also hold true: in other words, blocking 5HT2A receptors should promote dopamine release. Indeed, this is the case (see Figs. 2–23 and 2–24). When dopamine release is enhanced by an atypical antipsychotic via blockade of 5HT2A receptors, this allows the extra dopamine to compete with the atypical antipsychotic to reverse the blockade of D2 receptors (Fig. 2–24). Thus, 5HT2A antagonism reverses D2 antagonism in the nigrostriatal dopamine pathway. Not surprisingly, this leads to a

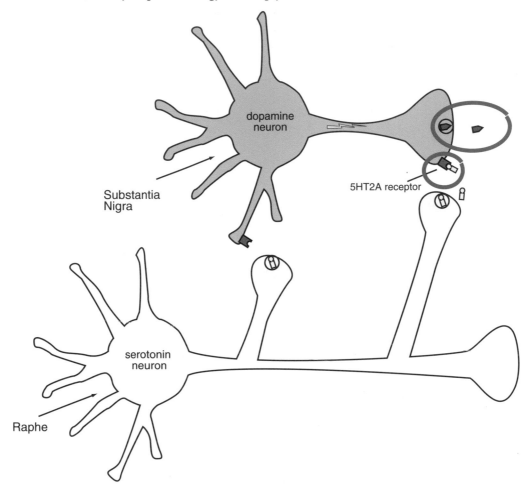

FIGURE 2–20. *Serotonin regulation of dopamine release from nigrostriatal dopamine neurons*, part 3. Here, serotonin is being released from a synaptic connection projection from axoaxonal contacts or by volume neurotransmission between serotoninergic axon terminals and dopamine axon terminals, resulting in serotonin occupying a postsynaptic serotonin 2A (5HT2A) receptor (*bottom red circle*). Because of this, dopamine release from its axonal terminal is now inhibited (*top red circle*).

reduction or even an absence of EPS and tardive dyskinesia, because there is a reduction of D2 receptor blockade in this pathway.

The serotonin-dopamine antagonism (SDA) properties of the atypical antipsychotics all exploit this ability of serotonin 2A antagonism to play a sort of indirect "tug-of-war" with dopamine 2 antagonism by causing dopamine release, which in turn mitigates or reverses dopamine 2 antagonism. Which one wins—D2 antagonism, or dopamine stimulation—depends on the drug (for conventional antipsychotics, D2 antagonism always wins), the dose (D2 antagonism is more likely to win at higher doses of atypical antipsychotics), and the pathway in the brain, as explained below.

In the nigrostriatal dopamine pathway, positron emission tomography (PET) scans document that atypical antipsychotics bind to fewer D2 receptors in the basal

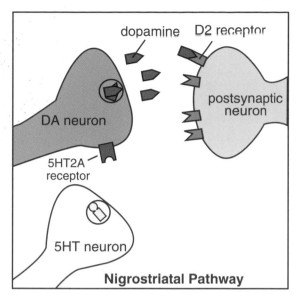

FIGURE 2–21. Enlarged view of **serotonin** (5HT) and **dopamine** (DA) interactions in the **nigrostriatal** dopamine pathway. Normally, serotonin inhibits dopamine release. In this figure, dopamine is being released because no serotonin is stopping it. Specifically, no serotonin is present at its 5HT2A receptor on the nigrostriatal dopaminergic neuron (but see Fig. 2–22).

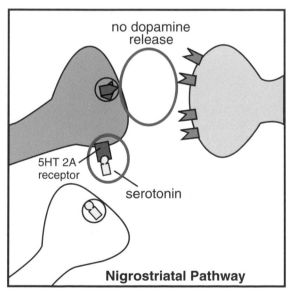

FIGURE 2–22. Now dopamine (DA) release is being **inhibited** by serotonin (5HT) in the nigrostriatal dopamine pathway. When serotonin occupies its 5HT2A receptor on the dopamine neuron (*lower red circle*), this inhibits dopamine release, so there is no dopamine in the synapse (*upper red circle*). Compare this with Figure 2–21.

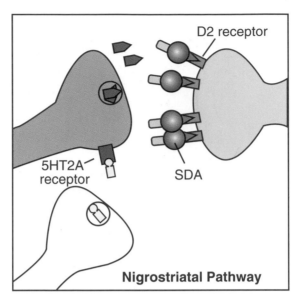

FIGURE 2–23. Here postsynaptic dopamine 2 receptors are being blocked by a serotonin-dopamine antagonist (SDA) atypical antipsychotic in the **nigrostriatal** dopamine pathway. This shows what would happen if only the dopamine 2 blocking action of an atypical antipsychotic were active—namely, the drug would only bind to postsynaptic D2 receptors and block them. However, see Figure 2–24.

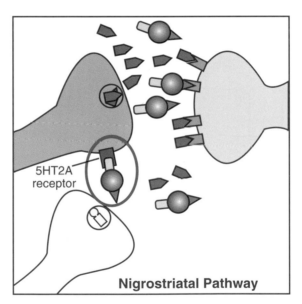

FIGURE 2–24. This figure shows how dopamine 2 (D2) receptor blockade is **reversed** by serotonin 2A receptor blockade in the **nigrostriatal** pathway. In contrast to Figure 2–23, this figure shows the dual action of the serotonin-dopamine antagonists (SDAs). Only the first action was shown in Figure 2–23, namely, binding to D2 receptors. The second action is shown here, namely, binding to serotonin 2A (5HT2A) receptors. The interesting thing is that this second action actually reverses the first. That is, blocking a 5HT2A receptor reverses the blockade of a D2 receptor. This happens because dopamine is released when serotonin can no longer inhibit its release. Another term for this is disinhibition. Thus, blocking a 5HT2A receptor disinhibits the dopamine neuron, causing dopamine to pour out of it. The consequence of this disinhibition is that the dopamine can then compete with the SDA for the D2 receptor and reverse the inhibition there. That is why **5HT2A blockers reverse D2 blockers in the striatum**. As D2 blockade is thereby reversed, SDAs cause little or no EPS or tardive dyskinesia.

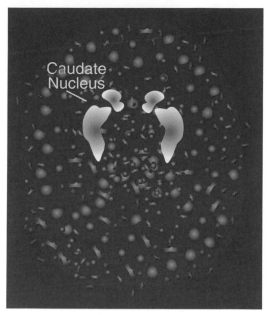

conventional antipsychotic

FIGURE 2–25. Artist's concept of a **conventional antipsychotic** drug binding to postsynaptic **dopamine 2 receptors** in the **nigrostriatal** pathway. Autoradiographic and radioreceptor labeling studies in experimental animals as well as positron emission tomography (PET) scans in schizophrenic patients have established that antipsychotic doses of conventional antipsychotic drugs essentially saturate the binding capacity of these receptors, Bright colors indicate binding to D2 receptors and show here that about 90% of dopamine receptors are being blocked at an antipsychotic dose of a conventional antipsychotic in a schizophrenic patient, which explains why such doses also cause EPS.

ganglia in schizophrenic patients than do conventional antipsychotics at matched antipsychotic efficacies (Figs. 2–25 and 2–26). Thus, about 90% of D2 receptors are blocked when a patient takes an antipsychotic dose of a conventional antipsychotic (Fig. 2–25), but less than 70 to 80% are blocked with an atypical antipsychotic (Fig. 2–26). This puts the threshold of D2 blockade below the level necessary to produce EPS in many patients. Thus, in the SDA tug-of-war in the nigrostriatal pathway, dopamine release is sufficient to reduce D2 antagonist binding just enough to create the best known atypical clinical feature of these agents, namely, reduced EPS without loss of antipsychotic efficacy. Thus, this is a win for dopamine release over dopamine blockade in the nigrostriatal tug-of-war.

The Mesocortical Pathway and the Pharmacology of Improved Negative Symptoms

Serotonin 2A antagonism not only reverses dopamine 2 antagonism but causes a net increase in dopamine activity in the mesocortical dopamine pathway, where the balance between serotonin and dopamine is different from that in the nigrostriatal dopamine pathway. That is, unlike the nigrostriatal dopamine pathway, in which dopamine 2 receptors predominate, there is a preponderance of serotonin 2A receptors over dopamine 2 receptors in many parts of the cerebral cortex. Thus, in the mesocortical dopamine pathway, atypical antipsychotics with SDA properties have

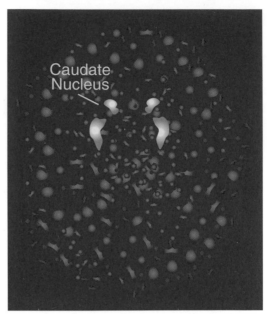

serotonin-dopamine antagonist

FIGURE 2–26. Artist's concept of an **atypical antipsychotic** drug binding to postsynaptic **dopamine 2 receptors** in the **nigrostriatal** pathway. Although this patient is receiving as much antipsychotic benefit as the patient in the previous scan (Fig. 2–25), the binding of drug to D2 receptors in the striatum is less intense in color, indicating only about 70 to 80% blockade of receptors. This reduction is sufficient to put the patient below the threshold for EPS. Thus, this patient has the benefit of the drug's antipsychotic actions, but no EPS. Presumably, blockade of D2 receptors in the mesolimbic dopamine pathway (not shown), which is the target for reducing positive symptoms of psychosis, is matched for both patients in Figures 2–25 and 2–26, which is why they both have relief of psychosis.

a more profound effect in blocking densely populated cortical serotonin 2A receptors, thereby increasing DA release, than in blocking thinly populated cortical D2 receptors. This results in considerable amounts of serotonin 2A antagonist binding and also of dopamine release, but not much dopamine 2 antagonism in this part of the brain. Bottom line? Dopamine release wins again over dopamine blockade in the mesocortical tug-of-war. Dopamine release in this part of the brain should be theoretically favorable for ameliorating negative symptoms of schizophrenia, and clinical trials show that atypical antipsychotics improve negative symptoms better than either placebo or conventional antipsychotics. Recall that dopamine deficiency in the mesocortical dopamine pathway is hypothesized to be one of the contributing causes of the negative symptoms of schizophrenia (Fig. 2–27). Thus, the nature of serotonin-dopamine antagonism in the mesocortical dopamine pathway has helped atypical antipsychotics to resolve the dilemma of how to increase theoretically deficient dopamine in the mesocortical dopamine pathway to treat negative symptoms and yet simultaneously to reduce theoretically hyperactive dopamine in the mesolimbic dopamine pathway to treat positive symptoms.

Positron emission tomography scans reveal that an antipsychotic dose of a conventional antipsychotic drug does not block serotonin 2A receptors in the cortex

Mesocortical Pathway

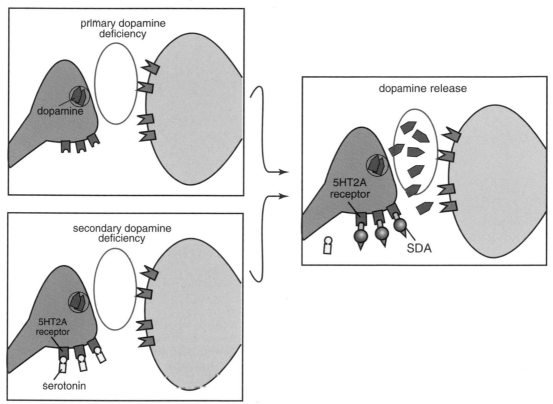

FIGURE 2–27. The **mesocortical** dopamine pathway may mediate deficits in **cognitive function-ing** and **negative symptoms** in schizophrenia because of a relative deficiency in dopamine, due either to a primary deficiency or to various secondary causes, such as serotonin excess. In either case, block-ade of 5HT2A receptors with an atypical antipsychotic should lead to dopamine release, which could compensate for the dopamine deficiency and improve negative and cognitive symptoms.

as expected, because these drugs lack such binding properties (Fig. 2–28), but that an antipsychotic dose of an atypical antipsychotic causes a nearly complete block-ade of the serotonin 2A receptors there (Fig. 2–29). Where serotonin 2A receptors are blocked, dopamine is being released (see Fig. 2–27), which explains in part why atypical antipsychotics improve negative symptoms better than do conventional antipsychotics. Clearly, other neurochemical mechanisms are operative in the patho-physiology of negative symptoms, but serotonin and dopamine may make an impor-tant contribution, as explained by these actions in the mesolimbic pathway.

The Tuberoinfundibular Pathway and the Pharmacology of Reduced Hyperprolactinemia

Serotonin 2A antagonism may reverse dopamine 2 antagonism in the tuberoin-fundibular pathway. There is an antagonistic and reciprocal relationship between serotonin and dopamine in the control of prolactin secretion from the pituitary

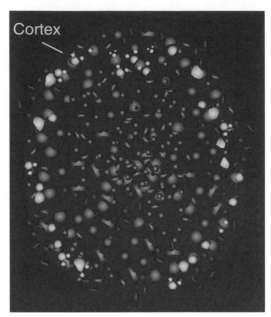

conventional antipsychotic

FIGURE 2–28. Artist's concept of a **conventional antipsychotic drug** binding to postsynaptic **serotonin 2A receptors** in the **cerebral cortex**, including mesocortical dopaminergic projections and dorsolateral prefrontal cortex. Autoradiographic and radioreceptor labeling studies in experimental animals as well as positron emission tomography (PET) scans in schizophrenic patients have established that antipsychotic doses of conventional antipsychotic drugs essentially bind to none of these receptors. Bright colors indicate binding to 5HT2A receptors, and the lack of any receptors lighting up here confirms the lack of binding to cortical 5HT2A receptors. Where cortical 5HT2A receptors are blocked, dopamine is being released. This patient is receiving an antipsychotic dose of a conventional antipsychotic, but there is no effect on 5HT2A receptors in the cortex because these drugs do not interact with 5HT2A receptors. See the contrast with Figure 2–29.

lactotroph cells. That is, dopamine inhibits prolactin release by stimulating D2 receptors (Fig. 2–30), whereas serotonin promotes prolactin release by stimulating 5HT2A receptors (Fig. 2–31).

Thus, when D2 receptors are blocked by a conventional antipsychotic, dopamine can no longer inhibit prolactin release, so prolactin levels rise (Fig. 2–32). However, in the case of an atypical antipsychotic, there is simultaneous inhibition of 5HT2A receptors, so serotonin can no longer stimulate prolactin release (Fig. 2–33). This tends to mitigate the hyperprolactinemia of D2 receptor blockade. Although this is interesting theoretical pharmacology, in practice not all serotonin-dopamine antagonists reduce prolactin secretion to the same extent, and some do not reduce it at all.

The Mesolimbic Pathway and the Pharmacology of Improved Positive Symptoms

Serotonin 2A antagonism fortunately fails to reverse D2 antagonism in the mesolimbic system. If serotonin 2A antagonism reverses, at least in part, the effects of D2 antagonism in several dopamine pathways, then why does it not reverse

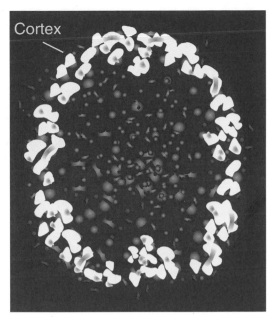

serotonin-dopamine antagonist

FIGURE 2–29. Artist's concept of an **atypical antipsychotic drug** binding to postsynaptic **serotonin 2A (5HT2A) receptors** in **cerebral cortex**, including mesocortical dopamine projections and dorsolateral prefrontal cortex. Autoradiographic and radioreceptor studies in animals as well as positron emission tomography (PET) scans in schizophrenic patients have established that 5HT2A receptors in the cortex are essentially saturated by antipsychotic doses of atypical antipsychotic drugs. Presumably, dopamine release occurs at the sites where there is 5HT2A binding, and that could lead to improvement in cognitive functioning and negative symptoms by a mechanism not possible for conventional antipsychotic agents (cf. Fig. 2–28).

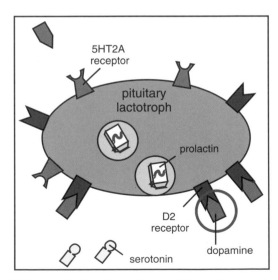

FIGURE 2–30. **Dopamine inhibits prolactin** release from pituitary lactotroph cells in the pituitary gland (*red circle*).

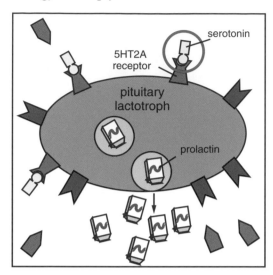

FIGURE 2–31. **Serotonin stimulates prolactin** release from pituitary lactotroph cells in the pituitary gland (*red circle*). Thus, serotonin and dopamine have a reciprocal regulatory action on prolactin release, and oppose each other's actions.

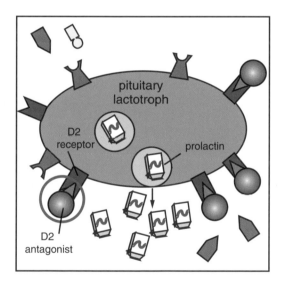

FIGURE 2–32. **Conventional antipsychotic drugs** are D2 antagonists and thus oppose dopamine's inhibitory role on prolactin secretion from pituitary lactotrophs. Therefore, drugs that block D2 receptors **increase prolactin** levels (*red circle*).

the antipsychotic actions of D2 blockade in the mesolimbic dopamine pathway? Evidently, the antagonism by serotonin of the effects of dopamine in this pathway is not robust enough to cause the reversal of D2 receptors by atypical antipsychotics or to mitigate the actions of atypical antipsychotics on positive symptoms of psychosis.

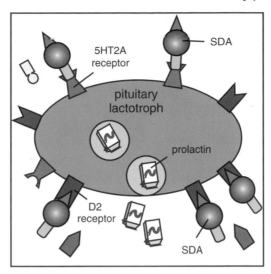

FIGURE 2–33. This figure shows how serotonin 2A antagonism **reverses** the ability of dopamine 2 (D2) antagonism to increase prolactin secretion. As **dopamine and serotonin have reciprocal regulatory roles** in the control of **prolactin** secretion, one cancels the other. Thus, stimulating 5HT2A receptors reverses the effects of stimulating D2 receptors (cf. Figs. 2–30 and 2–31). The same thing works in reverse, namely, blockade of 5HT2A receptors (shown here) reverses the effects of blocking D2 receptors (shown in Fig. 2–32).

Summary of Actions of Atypical Antipsychotics as a Class

In summary, for conventional antipsychotics dopamine blockade wins the tug-of-war in every dopamine pathway, resulting in antipsychotic actions for positive symptoms, but at a cost of worsened, or at least not improved, negative symptoms, production of EPS, tardive dyskinesia, and hyperprolactinemia. On the other hand, it appears that atypical antipsychotics let you "have your cake and eat it too," that is, dopamine blockade wins the all important tug-of-war over dopamine release where it must win to treat disruptive positive symptoms, namely, in the mesolimbic dopamine pathway. However, the very opposite is occurring simultaneously in the mesocortical dopamine pathway when an atypical antipsychotic is administered, since dopamine release wins the tug-of-war over dopamine blockade in that area of the brain, and negative symptoms are consequently improved, not worsened as they often are with conventional antipsychotics. The "icing" on the cake is that during atypical antipsychotic drug administration, dopamine release wins the tug-of-war over dopamine blockade both in the nigrostriatal and tuberoinfundibular dopamine pathways to an extent sufficient to reduce EPS and hyperprolactinemia as well, leading largely to elimination of these disabling side effects for many patients as compared with taking conventional antipsychotic drugs. This mix of favorable outcomes appears to be due largely to the differences between serotonin-dopamine antagonism in different parts of the brain, so that simultaneous blockade of D2 receptors and 5HT2A receptors can do nearly the opposite things in the same brain at the same time with the same drug!

Although there are obviously many other factors at play here and this is an overly simplistic explanation, it is a useful starting point for beginning to appreciate the pharmacological actions of atypical antipsychotics as a class of drugs.

Atypical Antipsychotics: Several Unique Drugs or One Class of Several Drugs?

Serotonin-dopamine antagonism is a key concept for explaining some of the atypical clinical actions of several atypical antipsychotics, but it is not a sufficient explanation for all the properties of these unique therapeutic agents. Some serotonin-dopamine antagonists do not have the atypical clinical properties of the five well-established atypical antipsychotics cited above (e.g., loxapine is a serotonin-dopamine antagonist but considered to be a conventional antipsychotic, especially at high doses). Also, some drugs (e.g., amisulpride) with low EPS are not necessarily serotonin-dopamine antagonists. Furthermore, some serotonin-dopamine antagonists at high doses begin to lose their atypical properties (e.g., risperidone). Thus, other pharmacologic and clinical factors must be considered to gain a full understanding of the several antipsychotics currently considered atypical. Here, we will consider five agents on an ever-expanding list of atypical antipsychotics: clozapine, risperidone, olanzapine, quetiapine, and ziprasidone. Several other candidates are considered in later sections as well.

In addition to the earlier limited definition of an atypical antipsychotic as an agent with serotonin 2A and dopamine 2 antagonist properties associated with decreased EPS, there are other pharmacologic properties associated with the five currently marketed atypical antipsychotics. Furthermore, no two agents have exactly identical properties, including multiple pharmacologic actions at serotonin and dopamine receptor subtypes in addition to SDA actions (e.g., D1, D3, and D4 as well as 5HT1A, 5HT1D, 5HT2C, 5HT3, 5HT6, and 5HT7) (Fig. 2–33) and multiple pharmacologic actions at other neurotransmitter receptors (such as alpha 1 and alpha 2 noradrenergic, muscarinic cholinergic, and histamine 1 receptors, as well as both the serotonin and norepinephrine reuptake pumps) (Fig. 2–34).

Not only do the atypical antipsychotics have incremental pharmacological actions beyond SDA actions, but they also have additional favorable and unfavorable clinical properties beyond the limited clinical definition of reduced EPS and actions on positive symptoms of psychosis. These additional favorable properties include the ability to improve negative symptoms in schizophrenic patients better than do conventional antipsychotics; the ability to cause little or no elevation of prolactin levels; the ability to improve positive symptoms in schizophrenic patients resistant to conventional antipsychotics; the ability to improve mood and reduce suicide not only in patients with schizophrenia but also in bipolar patients in manic, mixed, and depressed phases of their illnesses. Additional unfavorable clinical properties of atypical antipsychotics can include weight gain, sedation, seizures, or agranulocytosis.

Each of the major atypical antipsychotics differs on how well these various favorable and unfavorable clinical features have been established in large clinical trials. Furthermore, individual patients can have responses very different from the median response predicted from group outcomes of clinical trials, as well as very different responses to one of these agents as compared with another. In practice, therefore, the currently marketed agents in the atypical antipsychotic class can each be appreciated

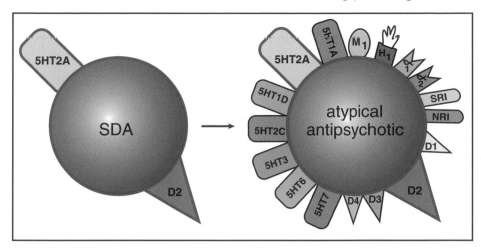

FIGURE 2–34. **Beyond the SDA concept.** Atypical antipsychotics are not merely simple serotonin-dopamine antagonists (SDAs). In truth, they have some of the most complex mixtures of pharmacologic properties in psychopharmacology. Shown here is an icon with all these properties. Beyond antagonism of serotonin 2A and dopamine 2 receptors, some agents in this class interact with multiple other receptor subtypes for both dopamine and serotonin, including 5HT1A, 5HT1D, 5HT2C, 5HT3, 5HT6, 5HT7, and D1, D3, and D4. Other neurotransmitter systems are involved as well, including both norepinephrine and serotonin reuptake blockade, as well as antimuscarinic, antihistaminic, and alpha 1 adrenergic plus alpha 2 adrenergic blockade. No two atypical antipsychotics, however, have identical binding properties, which probably helps to explain why they all have distinctive clinical properties.

as much for the differences they have from one another as for the pharmacological and clinical actions they share.

Although it is not yet clear why the various atypical antipsychotics differ from each other, the answer is most likely to be found in the pharmacologic properties, other than serotonin 2A dopamine–2 antagonism, that they do *not* share in common. Although some of these properties are still unknown, many of them are known (and are shown in Figure 2–34 and in the individual icons for the various atypical antipsychotics discussed later in this chapter). Of the 17 pharmacologic properties detailed in these icons, some undoubtedly mediate side effects, and others may mediate additional therapeutic actions mentioned here. This raises the question: Are atypical antipsychotics with multiple therapeutic mechanisms better than those with fewer therapeutic mechanisms (see Fig. 2–35)?

The idea of synergy among multiple pharmacologic mechanisms also forms the rationale for combining drugs of differing therapeutic actions in patients who do not respond to various antidepressants with single pharmacologic mechanisms. Could such a rationale also explain why one schizophrenic patient may sometimes respond to an atypical antipsychotic with one specific blend of multiple pharmacologic mechanisms better than to another atypical antipsychotic with a different mixture of such mechanisms? Head-to-head comparisons of atypical antipsychotics are only beginning to help develop a rational basis for choosing one atypical antipsychotic over another now that the superiority of this class of agents over conventional antipsychotics seems well established. Currently, the best atypical antipsychotic

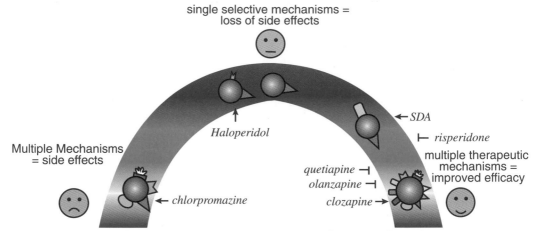

**Are Antipsychotics with Multiple Therapeutic Mechanisms Better
than Selective Dopamine 2 Antagonists?**

FIGURE 2–35. Are antipsychotics with **multiple therapeutic mechanisms** better than selective D2 antagonists or selective SDAs? The original phenothiazine antipsychotics are conceptualized as conventional antipsychotics with the desirable pharmacologic property of D2 antagonism, whereas their other pharmacologic properties are considered unwanted, and the cause of side effects (see left side of spectrum). Thus, when higher-potency D2 antagonists with lesser secondary pharmacologic properties were introduced, such as haloperidol, this was considered an advance (see middle of spectrum). During this era, the idea was that the most desirable agents were those with the greatest selectivity and with only one primary action, namely D2 antagonism. Next, in the SDA era, the concept was developed that, at a minimum, 5HT2A antagonism (SDA) should be combined with D2 antagonism to make a more efficacious, better tolerated antipsychotic, namely an atypical antipsychotic. Taking things a step further is the proposition that even greater efficacy can be attained with a further mix of pharmacologic properties, especially for treatment-refractory schizophrenia and for treating additional dimensions of symptoms in schizophrenia beyond positive and negative symptoms, such as mood and cognition symptoms.

for an individual patient is often discovered by trial and error. Because differences among the drugs in this class can be important, a brief discussion of each of the five agents currently in clinical use is included here. Other specific agents will be discussed in later sections of this chapter.

Clozapine

Clozapine is considered to be the prototype of the atypical antipsychotics, as it was the first to be recognized as having few if any extrapyramidal side effects, not causing tardive dyskinesia, and not elevating prolactin. Clozapine is one of five antipsychotics with somewhat related chemical structures (Fig. 2–36). Although certainly a serotonin 2A–dopamine 2 antagonist, clozapine also has one of the most complex pharmacologic profiles in psychopharmacology, let alone among the atypical antipsychotics (Fig. 2–37).

Clozapine is the one atypical antipsychotic recognized as particularly effective when conventional antipsychotic agents have failed. Although patients may occasionally experience an "awakening" (in the Oliver Sachs sense), characterized by

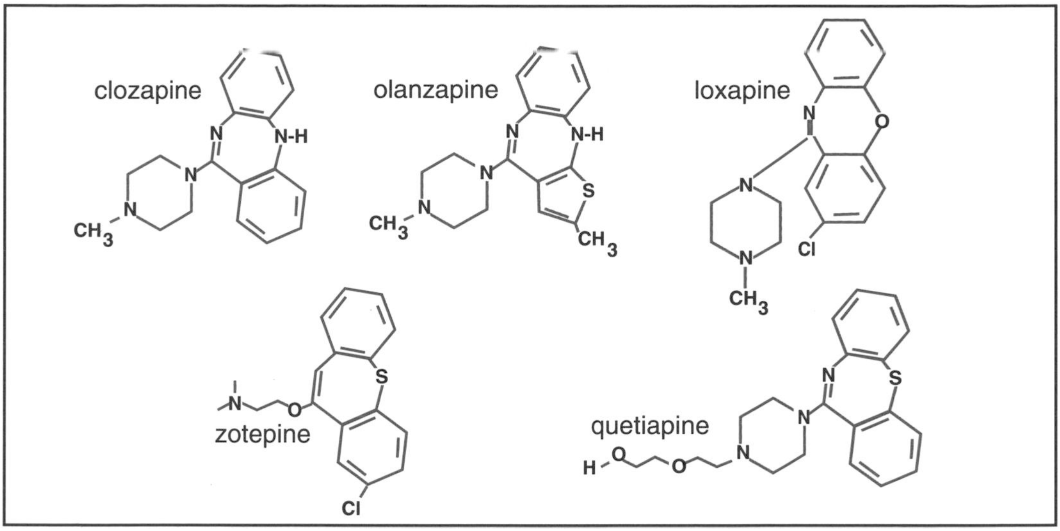

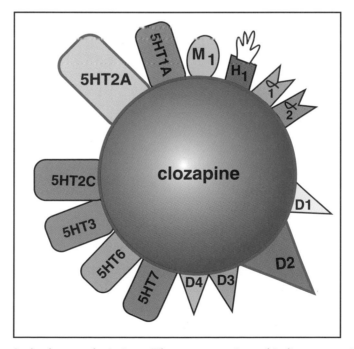

FIGURE 2–36. Structural **formulas** for **clozapine** and four other antipsychotics, namely, **olanzapine, quetiapine, loxapine, and zotepine**. Interestingly, all five of these are also SDAs, but not all of them appear to be atypical antipsychotics (e.g., loxapine is conventional, and zotepine is still being characterized). Also, clinical properties and pharmacological characteristics vary considerably among those that are clearly atypical (i.e., clozapine, olanzapine, and quetiapine).

FIGURE 2–37. **Clozapine**'s pharmacologic icon. The most prominent binding properties of clozapine are represented here; it has perhaps one of the most complex binding portfolios in psychopharmacology. Its binding properties vary greatly with technique and species and from one laboratory to another. This icon portrays a qualitative consensus of current thinking about the binding properties of clozapine, which are constantly being revised and updated.

return to a near normal level of cognitive, interpersonal, and vocational functioning and not just significant improvement in positive symptoms of psychosis, this is unfortunately quite rare. The fact that it can be observed at all, however, gives hope to the possibility that a state of wellness might some day be achieved in schizophrenia by the right mix of pharmacologic mechanisms. Such awakenings have been observed on rare occasions in association with treatment with other atypical antipsychotics as well, but rarely if ever in association with conventional antipsychotic treatment.

Clozapine is also the only antipsychotic drug associated with the risk of a life-threatening and occasionally fatal complication called *agranulocytosis* which occurs in 0.5 to 2% of patients. Because of this, patients must have their blood counts monitored weekly for the first 6 months of treatment and then every 2 weeks for as long as they are treated. Clozapine also entails an increased risk of seizures, especially at high doses. It can be very sedating and is associated with the greatest degree of weight gain among the antipsychotics. Thus, clozapine may have the greatest efficacy but the most side effects among the atypical antipsychotics.

Pharmacologists have been attempting to define what it is about clozapine's biochemical mechanism of action that accounts for its special efficacy as well as its side effects. As discussed extensively in this chapter, SDA properties may account in part for reducing EPS, for reducing tardive dyskinesia, and perhaps even for lack of prolactin elevation; SDA properties may even help explain improvement in negative symptoms of schizophrenia. However, the concept of SDA does not appear to explain the therapeutic actions of clozapine in treatment-resistant cases because clozapine is superior to other agents that share this property.

Serotonin-dopamine antagonist properties also do not explain clozapine's side effects of weight gain, sedation, seizures, and agranulocytosis. The mechanism of clozapine's induction of agranulocytosis remains unclear, but fortunately no other atypical antipsychotic drug appears to share this problem. Seizures are also poorly understood but are not a serious problem for any other atypical antipsychotic. Weight gain, most notorious for clozapine among all of the atypical antipsychotics, appears to correlate best with its antihistaminic binding properties, perhaps made worst by concomitant serotonin 2C antagonist actions. Sedation may be linked to antihistaminic and anticholinergic actions.

In view of the risk/benefit ratio for clozapine, this agent is not generally considered a first-line agent for the treatment of psychosis but one to consider when several other agents have failed. It is especially useful in quelling violence and aggression in difficult patients, may reduce suicide rates in schizophrenia, and may reduce tardive dyskinesia severity, especially over long treatment intervals.

Risperidone

This agent has a different chemical structure (Fig. 2–38) and a considerably simpler pharmacologic profile than clozapine (Fig. 2–39). Risperidone is especially atypical at lower doses but can become more "conventional" at high doses in that EPS can occur if the dose is too high. Risperidone thus has favored uses, not only in schizophrenia at moderate doses but also for conditions in which low doses of conventional antipsychotics have been used in the past, for example, for elderly patients with psychosis, agitation, and behavioral disturbances associated with dementia and

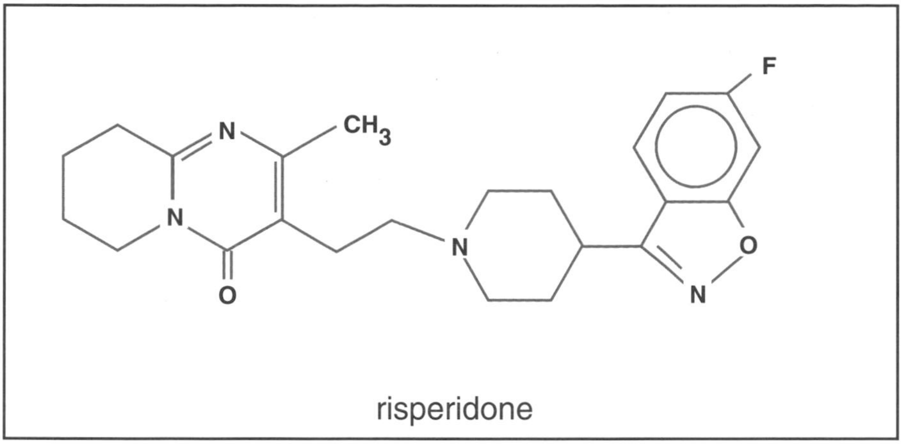

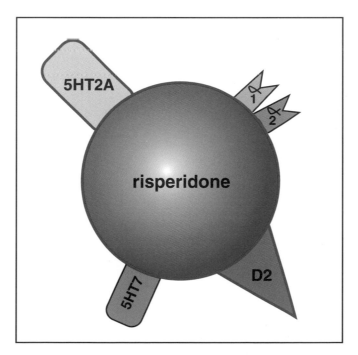

FIGURE 2–38. Structural **formula** of **risperidone**.

FIGURE 2–39. **Risperidone**'s pharmacologic icon, portraying a qualitative consensus of current thinking about the binding properties of this drug. Among the atypical antipsychotics, it has one of the simplest pharmacologic profiles and comes closest to an SDA. As with all atypical antipsychotics discussed in this chapter, binding properties vary greatly with technique and species and from one laboratory to another; they are constantly being revised and updated.

for children and adolescents with psychotic disorders. Although risperidone is an SDA, for reasons that are not clear it elevates prolactin to the same degree as conventional antipsychotics, even at low doses.

Many studies show that risperidone is a highly effective agent for positive symptoms of schizophrenia and also improves negative symptoms of schizophrenia better than do conventional antipsychotics. Early studies show a very low incidence of tardive dyskinesia with long-term use and also show that some patients improve on risperidone when conventional antipsychotics fail, although probably not as well as they would on clozapine. Ongoing studies suggest that risperidone may improve cognitive functioning not only in schizophrenia, but also in dementias, such as Alzheimer's disease. Risperidone may also improve mood in schizophrenia and in both the manic and depressed phases of bipolar disorder. There is less weight gain with risperidone than with some other atypical antipsychotic agents, perhaps because risperidone does not block histamine 1 receptors, but weight gain is still a problem for some patients.

Olanzapine

Although olanzapine has a chemical structure related to that of clozapine (Fig. 2–36), it is more potent than clozapine and has several differentiating pharmacologic (Fig. 2–40) and clinical features, not only as compared with clozapine (Fig. 2–37) but also as compared with risperidone (Fig. 2–39). Olanzapine is atypical in that it generally lacks EPS, not only at moderate doses but usually even at high doses. Thus, olanzapine tends to be used for some of the most difficult cases of schizophrenia, bipolar disorder, and other types of psychosis in which good control of psychosis without EPS is still desired, yet aggressive treatment is required. On the other hand, this approach can be very expensive.

Olanzapine lacks the extreme sedating properties of clozapine but can be somewhat sedating. Olanzapine is associated with weight gain, perhaps because of its antihistaminic and serotonin 2C antagonist properties (Fig. 2–40). Olanzapine does not often raise prolactin. Early studies suggest a very low incidence of tardive dyskinesia with long-term use and also suggest that some patients improve with olanzapine when conventional antipsychotics fail, although probably not as much as they would with clozapine. Many studies demonstrate that olanzapine is highly effective for positive symptoms of schizophrenia and also improves negative symptoms of schizophrenia better than do conventional antipsychotics. Ongoing studies also show that olanzapine improves mood, not only in schizophrenia but also in the manic and depressed phases of bipolar disorder, suggesting that it may be a first-line treatment for bipolar disorder. Some studies suggest that olanzapine may improve cognitive functioning in schizophrenia and in dementia.

Quetiapine

Quetiapine also has a chemical structure related to that of clozapine (Fig. 2–36), but it has several differentiating pharmacologic (Fig. 2–41) and clinical features, not only as compared with clozapine (Fig. 2–37) but also as compared with risperidone (Fig. 2–39) and olanzapine (Fig. 2–40). Quetiapine is very atypical in that it causes virtually no EPS at any dose and no prolactin elevations. Thus, quetiapine

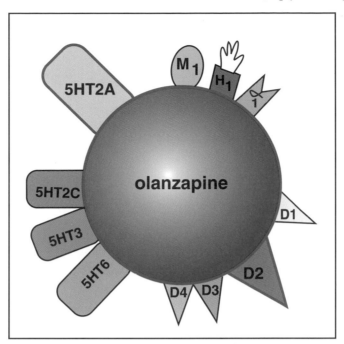

FIGURE 2–40. **Olanzapine**'s pharmacologic icon, portraying a qualitative consensus of current thinking about the binding properties of this drug. It has a complex pharmacology overlapping, yet different from, that of clozapine. As with all atypical antipsychotics discussed in this chapter, binding properties vary greatly with technique and species and from one laboratory to another; they are constantly being revised and updated.

tends to be the preferred atypical antipsychotic for patients with Parkinson's disease and psychosis. It is also useful in schizophrenia, bipolar disorder, and other types of psychosis, in which it has few extrapyramidal side effects.

Quetiapine can cause some weight gain, as it blocks histamine 1 receptors. It has shown species-specific inhibition of cholesterol biosynthesis in the lens of some animals, where it can cause cataracts, but is not documented to do this in humans. Some patients improve on quetiapine when conventional antipsychotics fail, although probably not as well as on clozapine. Studies demonstrate that quetiapine is highly effective for the positive symptoms and also improves the negative symptoms of schizophrenia. Ongoing studies are beginning to show that quetiapine may improve mood in schizophrenia and in the manic and depressed phases of bipolar disorder. Some studies suggest that quetiapine may improve cognitive functioning in schizophrenia and also in dementia.

Ziprasidone

Ziprasidone has a novel chemical structure (Fig. 2–42) and a quite novel pharmacological profile as compared with the other atypical antipsychotics (Fig. 2–43). Ziprasidone appears to be atypical, like the other agents in this class, in that it has low EPS and causes little or no prolactin elevation. Its major differentiating feature within this class may be that it seems to have little or no propensity to cause

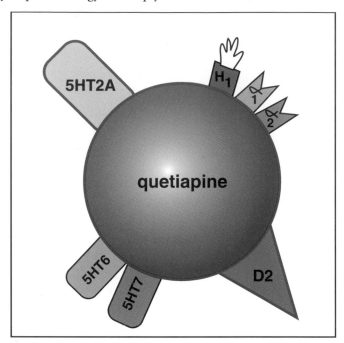

FIGURE 2–41. **Quetiapine**'s pharmacologic icon, portraying a qualitative consensus of current thinking about the binding properties of this drug. It has a unique pharmacological profile, different from those of all other atypical antipsychotics. As with all atypical antipsychotics discussed in this chapter, binding properties vary greatly with technique and species and from one laboratory to another; they are constantly being revised and updated.

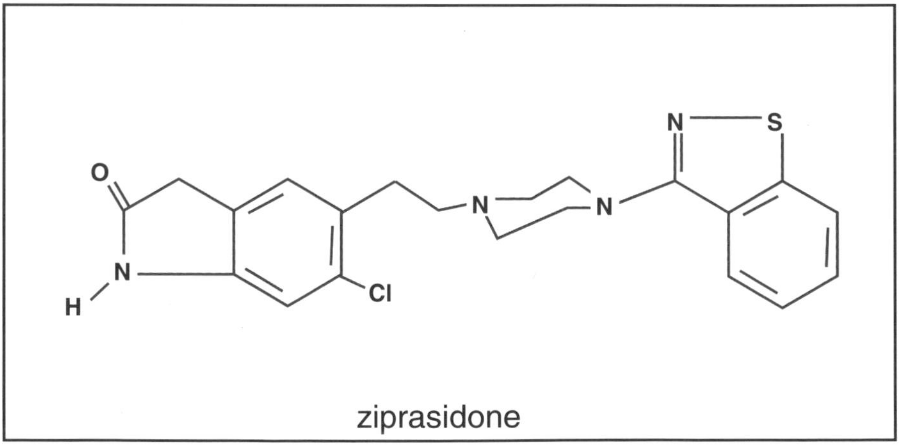

FIGURE 2–42. Structural **formula** of **ziprasidone**.

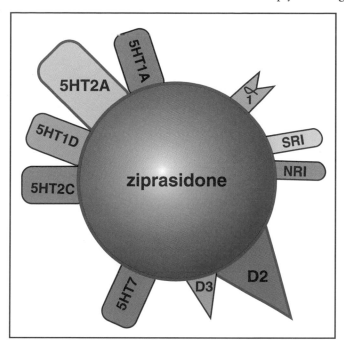

FIGURE 2–43. **Ziprasidone**'s pharmacologic icon, portraying a qualitative consensus of current thinking about the binding properties of this drug. It is the only atypical antipsychotic with 5HT1D antagonist and serotonin-norepinephrine reuptake blocking properties. As with all atypical antipsychotics discussed in this chapter, binding properties vary greatly with technique and species and from one laboratory to another; they are constantly being revised and updated.

weight gain, perhaps because it has no antihistaminic properties, although it does have serotonin 2C antagonist actions. Also, ziprasidone is the only atypical antipsychotic that is a serotonin 1D antagonist, a serotonin 1A agonist, and also inhibits both serotonin and norepinephrine reuptake. These latter pharmacologic actions would be expected to be both proserotonergic and pronoradrenergic, which might contribute to ziprasidone's favorable behavior as concerns weight but would predict antidepressant and anxiolytic actions as well. Antidepressant actions are being actively tested in schizophrenia and bipolar disorder to determine whether ziprasidone's theoretically advantageous pharmacological features will be demonstrable in head-to-head comparisons with other atypical antipsychotic agents.

Some patients improve with ziprasidone when conventional antipsychotics fail, although probably not as much as with clozapine. Studies demonstrate that ziprasidone is highly effective for the positive symptoms and also improves the negative symptoms of schizophrenia. Some studies suggest that ziprasidone may improve cognitive functioning in schizophrenia and also in dementia.

Pharmacokinetic Considerations for the Atypical Antipsychotic Drugs

Here we will discuss some specific pharmacokinetic issues relating to antipsychotic drugs.

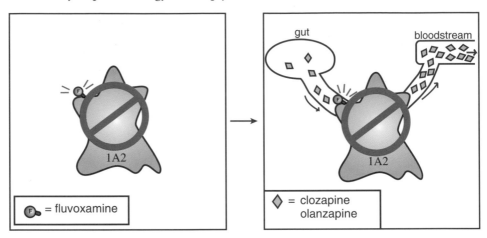

FIGURE 2–44. Clozapine and olanzapine are **substrates** for cytochrome **P450 1A2** (CYP450 1A2). When these drugs are given with an inhibitor of this enzyme, such as the antidepressant fluvoxamine, plasma levels of olanzapine and clozapine can rise.

Cytochrome P450 1A2

Recall that one of the key drug-metabolizing enzymes is the cytochrome P450 (CYP450) enzyme called 1A2. Two atypical antipsychotic drugs are substrates of 1A2, namely olanzapine and clozapine. That means that when they are given concomitantly with an inhibitor of this enzyme, such as the antidepressant fluvoxamine, their levels could rise (Fig. 2–44). Although this may not be particularly clinically important for olanzapine (other than causing slightly increased sedation), it could potentially raise plasma levels sufficiently in the case of clozapine to increase the risk of seizures. Thus, the dose of clozapine may need to be lowered when administering it with fluvoxamine, or another antidepressant may need to be chosen.

On the other hand, when an inducer of 1A2 is given concomitantly with either of the two antipsychotic substrates of 1A2, the level of the antipsychotic may fall. This happens when a patient begins to smoke, because smoking induces 1A2, and this would cause levels of olanzapine and clozapine to fall (Fig. 2–45). Theoretically this might cause patients stabilized on an antipsychotic dose to relapse if the levels fell too low. Also, cigarette smokers may require higher doses of these atypical antipsychotics than nonsmokers.

Cytochrome P450 2D6

Another cytochrome P450 enzyme of importance to atypical antipsychotic drugs is 2D6. Risperidone, clozapine, and olanzapine are all substrates for this enzyme (Fig. 2–46). Risperidone's metabolite is also an active atypical antipsychotic (Fig. 2–47), but the metabolites of clozapine and olanzapine are not. Recall that some antidepressants are inhibitors of CYP450 2D6 and thus can raise the levels of these three atypical antipsychotics (Fig. 2–48). For risperidone the clinical significance of this is uncertain, since both the parent drug and the metabolite are active. Theoretically, the dose of olanzapine and clozapine may have to be lowered when given with an antidepressant that blocks 2D6, although this is not often necessary in practice.

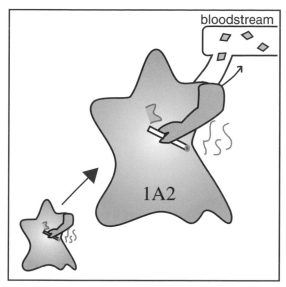

FIGURE 2–45. **Cigarette smoking**, quite common among schizophrenics, can induce the enzyme **CYP450 1A2** and lower the concentration of drugs metabolized by this enzyme, such as olanzapine and clozapine. Smokers may also require higher doses of these drugs than nonsmokers.

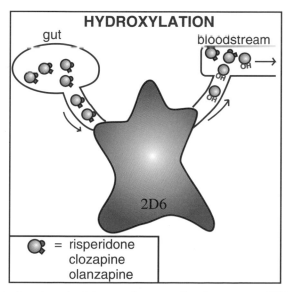

FIGURE 2–46. Several atypical antipsychotics are **substrates** for the enzyme **CYP450 2D6**, including risperidone, clozapine, and olanzapine.

Cytochrome P450 3A4

The CYP450 enzyme 3A4 metabolizes several atypical antipsychotics, including clozapine, quetiapine, ziprasidone, and sertindole (Fig. 2–49). Several psychotropic drugs are weak inhibitors of this enzyme, including the antidepressants fluvoxamine,

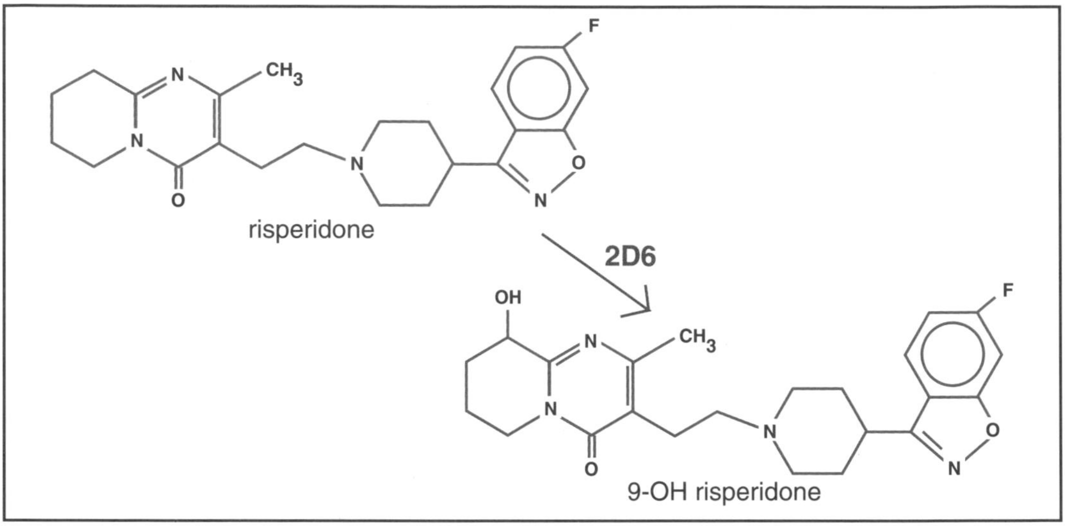

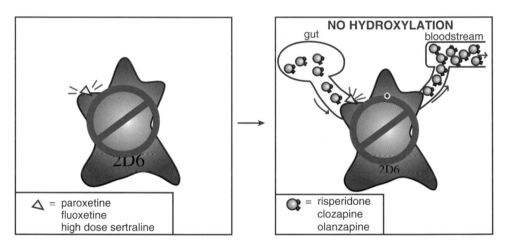

FIGURE 2–47. **Risperidone** is converted to an **active metabolite** by the enzyme CYP450 2D6.

FIGURE 2–48. Several antidepressants are **inhibitors** of **CYP450 2D6** and could theoretically raise the levels of 2D6 substrates such as risperidone, olanzapine, and clozapine. However, this is not usually clinically significant.

nefazodone, and norfluoxetine, which is an active metabolite of fluoxetine. Several nonpsychotropic drugs are powerful inhibitors of 3A4, including ketoconazole (antifungal), protease inhibitors (for human immunodeficiency virus (HIV) infections), and erythromycin (antibiotic). For the four atypical antipsychotics that are metabolized by 3A4, the clinical implication is that concomitant administration with a 3A4 inhibitor may require dosage reduction of the atypical antipsychotic (Fig. 2–50).

Drugs can not only be substrates for a cytochrome P450 enzyme or an inhibitor of a P450 enzyme, they can also be inducers of a cytochrome P450 enzyme and

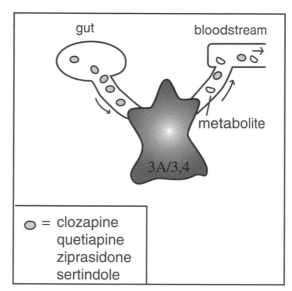

FIGURE 2–49. Several atypical antipsychotics are **substrates** for **CYP450 3A4**, including clozapine, quetiapine, ziprasidone, and sertindole.

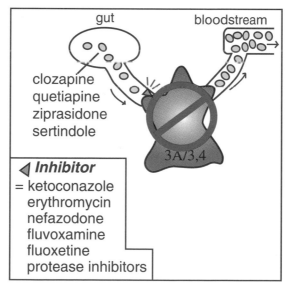

FIGURE 2–50. There are several **inhibitors** of **CYP450 3A4** that may increase levels of some atypical antipsychotics. The inhibitors are shown here, and the atypical antipsychotics including clozapine, quetiapine, ziprasidone, and sertindole, are shown as well.

thereby increase the activity of that enzyme. Since mood stabilizers may be frequently mixed with atypical antipsychotics, it is possible that carbamazepine may be added to the regimen of a patient previously stabilized on clozapine, quetiapine, ziprasidone, or sertindole. If so, the doses of these atypical antipsychotics may need to be increased over time to compensate for the induction of 3A4 by carbamazepine.

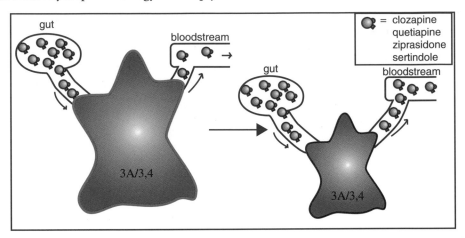

gut

bloodstream

gut

bloodstream

Q = clozapine
quetiapine
ziprasidone
sertindole

3A/3,4

3A/3,4

FIGURE 2–51. The enzyme **CYP450 3A4** can be **induced** by the anticonvulsant and mood stabilizer carbamazepine. If this agent is stopped in a patient who is receiving an atypical antipsychotic that is a substrate for this same enzyme (i.e., clozapine, quetiapine, ziprasidone, or sertindole), the doses of these antipsychotics may need to be reduced because the autoinduction of 3A4 by carbamazepine will reverse over time once it is discontinued.

On the other hand, if carbamazepine is stopped in a patient receiving one of these four atypical antipsychotics, the antipsychotic dose may need to be reduced, because the autoinduction of 3A4 by carbamazepine will reverse over time (Fig. 2–51).

Atypical Antipsychotics in Clinical Practice

The atypical antipsychotics are still relatively new, particularly some members. Information about new drugs is first available from clinical trials and then modified by observations from clinical practice, and the atypical antipsychotics are no exception to this pattern. Some findings from clinical practice have already confirmed those from clinical trials for the three marketed atypical antipsychotics (i.e., risperidone, olanzapine, and quetiapine) and are generally applicable to choosing an atypical antipsychotic for patients with a wide variety of psychotic disorders, although least is known about ziprasidone, the newest member of this group.

There are four main favorable findings.

First, atypical antipsychotics undoubtedly cause far fewer EPS than do conventional antipsychotics and often cause essentially no EPS (i.e., they really do perform in this respect, as predicted pharmacologically and as advertised). Second, atypical antipsychotics reduce negative symptoms of schizophrenia better than do conventional antipsychotics, but this may be because they do not make things worse as much as because they really reduce negative symptoms. The magnitude of this effect is not as robust as the effects on EPS, and further innovations will be necessary to solve the negative symptom problem in schizophrenia—nevertheless, this is a good start. Third, atypical antipsychotics reduce affective symptoms in schizophrenia and related disorders such as treatment-resistant depression and in bipolar disorder, where treatment effects appear to be quite robust. Fourth, atypical antipsychotics may possibly reduce cognitive symptoms in schizophrenia and related disorders such as Alzheimer's disease.

The magnitude of these properties is far from trivial and, in fact, makes the four atypical antipsychotics risperidone, olanzapine, quetiapine, and ziprasidone easily preferable as first-line therapies for psychosis, with conventional antipsychotics and clozapine as second-line therapies.

On the other hand, not everything that is suggested from controlled clinical trials of restricted populations of patients undergoing studies in ideal situations turns out to be applicable in the real world of clinical practice. Some of the perceptions from longer-term experience deriving from clinical practice that differ from the early indications arising from clinical trials may be summarized as follows.

First, different atypical antipsychotics can have clinically distinctive effects in different patients, unlike conventional antipsychotics, which mostly have the same clinical effects in different patients. Thus, median clinical effects in clinical trials may not be the best indicator of the range of clinical responses possible for individual patients. Second, optimal doses suggested from clinical trials often do not match optimal doses used in clinical practice, being too high for some drugs and too low for others. Third, atypical antipsychotics may not work as fast as conventional antipsychotics for acutely psychotic, aggressive, agitated patients requiring sedation and onset of action within minutes; for such patients, conventional antipsychotics or sedating benzodiazepines may be useful as adjuncts or as substitutes. Finally, although virtually all studies are head-to-head comparisons of monotherapies and/or placebo, many patients receive two antipsychotic drugs in clinical settings. Sometimes this is rational and justified, but often it is not.

Use of Atypical Antipsychotics for Positive Symptoms of Schizophrenia and Related Disorders

Although the usefulness of the atypical antipsychotics is best documented for the positive symptoms of schizophrenia, numerous studies are documenting the utility of these agents for the treatment of positive symptoms associated with several other disorders (discussed in Chapter 1; see Fig. 1–2). Atypical antipsychotics have become first-line acute and maintenance treatments for positive symptoms of psychosis, not only in schizophrenia but also in the acute manic and mixed manic-depressed phases of bipolar disorder; in depressive psychosis and schizoaffective disorder; in psychosis associated with behavioral disturbances in cognitive disorders such as Alzheimer's disease, Parkinson's disease, and other organic psychoses; and in psychotic disorders in children and adolescents (Fig. 2–52, first-line treatments). In fact, current treatment standards have evolved in many countries so that atypical antipsychotics have largely replaced conventional antipsychotics for the treatment of positive psychotic symptoms except in a few specific clinical situations.

One area of continuing use for conventional antipsychotics is in an especially acute setting with an uncooperative patient, where a drug with not only a rapid onset of action but also an intramuscular dosage formulation may be preferred (Fig. 2–52, in case of emergency). In practice, this can mean using sedating benzodiazepines as well as a few of the old-fashioned conventional antipsychotics available for intramuscular administration, such as haloperidol and loxapine. Several atypical antipsychotics are in the late testing stages for acute and chronic intramuscular administration.

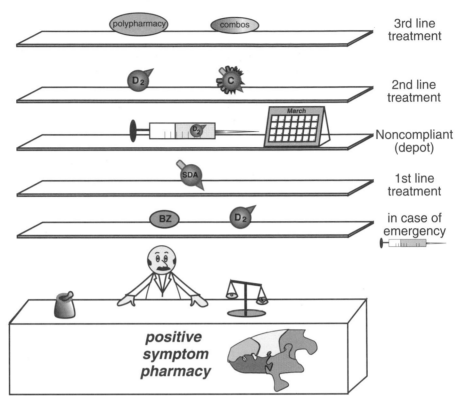

FIGURE 2–52. **Positive symptom pharmacy**. First-line treatment of positive symptoms is now atypical antipsychotics (SDA), not only for schizophrenia but also for positive symptoms associated with bipolar disorder, Alzheimer's disease, childhood psychoses, and other psychotic disorders. However, conventional antipsychotics (D2) and benzodiazepines (BZ) are still useful for acute intramuscular administration (in case of emergency), and D2 for monthly depot injections for noncompliant patients, as well as for second-line use after several atypical agents fail. Clozapine (C), polypharmacy, and combinations (combos) are relegated to second- and third-line treatment for positive symptoms of psychosis.

Another area of continuing use of conventional antipsychotics is for the non-compliant patient who may require monthly injections of a depot antipsychotic. No atypical antipsychotic is yet available for depot administration, although such formulations are under development. Otherwise, most clinicians generally try several different atypical antipsychotics before resorting to a trial of clozapine (with its encumbrance of weekly or biweekly blood counts), conventional antipsychotics, or various combination therapies of atypical antipsychotics with other agents (Fig. 2–52 second- and third-line treatments).

Use of Atypical Antipsychotics to Treat Disorders of Mood in Schizophrenia and Related Disorders

Profound mood-stabilizing effects of the atypical antipsychotic drugs were observed once their antipsychotic effects were documented. These effects on mood appear to be quite independent of their effects on positive symptoms of psychosis. The

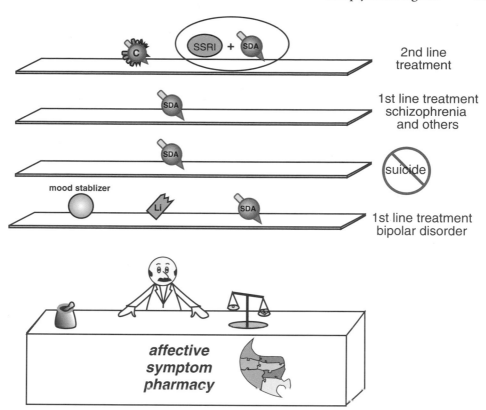

FIGURE 2–53. **Affective symptom pharmacy**. Atypical antipsychotics (SDA) are surprisingly effective in stabilizing mood in a number of disorders and are now becoming first-line treatments not only for psychotic symptoms of bipolar disorder (see positive symptom pharmacy in Fig. 2–52), but also for stabilizing manic, mixed, rapid cycling, and treatment-resistant mood states in bipolar patients (first-line treatment). Atypical agents may even reduce suicide rates among schizophrenic patients as well as bipolar disorder patients and improve mood and anxiety, even depression, in a number of disorders other than major depression. Atypical antipsychotics are also employed as adjuncts to antidepressants in treatment-resistant cases of nonpsychotic unipolar depression (second-line treatment). (Li is lithuim; C is clozapine; SSRI is serotonin selective reuptake inhibitor.)

most dramatic story may be how impressive the atypical antipsychotics are turning out to be for the treatment of bipolar disorder (Fig. 2–53). Although the best documented effect of these drugs is to reduce psychotic symptoms in the acute manic phase of bipolar disorder, it is clear that these agents also stabilize mood and can help in some of the most difficult cases, such as those marked by rapid cycling and mixed simultaneous manic-depressed states that are often nonresponsive to mood stabilizers and worsened by antidepressants. The atypical antipsychotics can help stabilize such patients for maintenance treatment, reduce the need for destabilizing antidepressants, and help boost the efficacy of concomitantly administered mood stabilizers.

Mood symptoms of depression are associated with many conditions in addition to major depressive disorder, including mood and anxiety symptoms in schizophrenia,

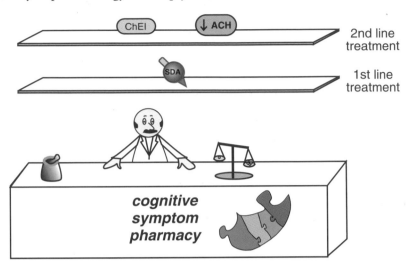

FIGURE 2–54. **Cognitive symptom pharmacy**. Atypical antipsychotic drugs (SDA) may improve cognitive functions in both schizophrenic and Alzheimer patients (first-line treatment). They may boost the actions of cholinesterase inhibitors (ChEIs) in Alzheimer's disease. It may also be useful to discontinue any anticholinergic medication that you can, a welcome bonus when switching from conventional antipsychotics to atypical antipsychotics (decreased A Ch).

schizoaffective disorder, bipolar manic/depressed/mixed/rapid cycling states, organic mood disorders, psychotic depression, childhood and adolescent mood disorders, treatment-resistant mood disorders, and many more (see Chapter 1, Fig. 1–6). Atypical antipsychotics are enjoying expanded use for the treatment of symptoms of depression and anxiety in schizophrenia that are troublesome but not severe enough to reach the diagnostic threshold for a major depressive episode or anxiety disorder; in these cases the antipsychotics are used not only to reduce such symptoms but hopefully also to reduce suicide rates, which are so high in schizophrenia (Fig. 2–53). Atypical antipsychotics may also be useful adjunctive treatments to antidepressants for unipolar depressed, nonpsychotic patients when several other antidepressants have failed.

Use of Atypical Antipsychotics for Cognitive Symptoms of Schizophrenia and Related Disorders

The severity of cognitive symptoms correlates with the long-term prognosis of schizophrenia. Cognitive symptoms clearly are a dimension of psychopathology that cuts across many disorders in psychiatry and neurology (see Chapter 1; Fig. 1–4). The atypical antipsychotics may improve cognition in several of these disorders and do this independently of their ability to reduce positive symptoms of psychosis (Fig. 2–54). In schizophrenia, there may be improvements in verbal fluency, serial learning, and executive functioning. In Alzheimer's disease, there may be improvements in memory and behavior, which could be additive or even synergistic with the improvement attained with concomitant treatment with other types of cognitive enhancers, such as the cholinesterase inhibitors. Much work is ongoing to see how

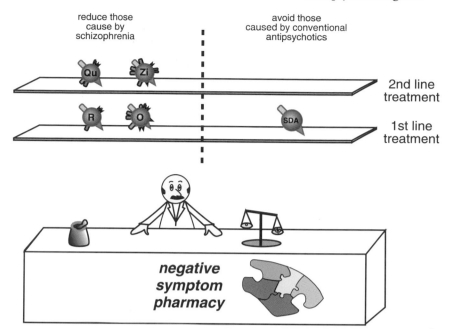

FIGURE 2–55. **Negative symptom pharmacy.** Negative symptoms can be improved in schizophrenia, both by switching from conventional antipsychotics, which make these symptoms worse, to atypical antipsychotics (SDA) that do not (right-hand side of pharmacy) or by the direct effects of atypical antipsychotics that boost negative symptoms. Olanzapine (O) and risperidone (R) both improve negative symptoms in schizophrenics better than do haloperidol or placebo in head-to-head trials (first line treatments). Ziprasidone (Zi) and quetiapine (Qu) so far both improve negative symptoms in schizophrenics as well as haloperidol and better than placebo in head-to-head trials (second-line treatments).

treatment with atypical antipsychotics can optimize cognitive function in schizophrenia and related disorders.

Use of Atypical Antipsychotics for Negative Symptoms of Schizophrenia

The negative symptoms of schizophrenia are thought to constitute a particularly unique feature, although certain aspects of these symptoms can overlap with symptoms that are not unique to schizophrenia itself (see Chapter 1 and Fig. 1–3). Any improvement in negative symptoms that can be gained from treatment with atypical antipsychotics is very important because the long-term outcome of schizophrenia is more closely correlated with severity of negative symptoms than it is with the severity of positive symptoms. However, it is already clear that significantly more robust treatment effects will be necessary than those offered by atypical antipsychotics if such symptoms are to be eliminated in the vast majority of schizophrenic patients. Nevertheless, there are two approaches to improving negative symptoms in the short run. First, negative symptoms secondary to conventional antipsychotics can be readily reduced by substituting an atypical antipsychotic (Fig. 2–55). Second, atypical antipsychotics actually improve negative symptoms. Olanzapine and risperidone have already documented better negative symptom

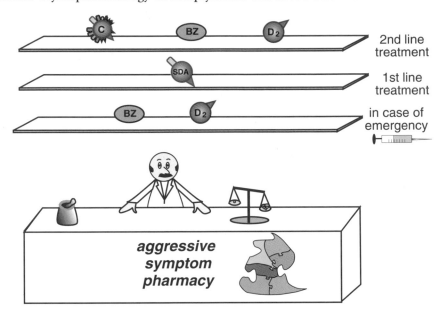

FIGURE 2–56. **Aggressive symptom pharmacy**. Atypical antipsychotics (SDA), when sufficiently effective, are preferable (first line) to conventional antipsychotics (D2) for the management of aggression, hostility, and impulse control because of their more favorable side effect profiles. However, in an acute situation, intramuscular conventional antipsychotics or benzodiazepines (BZ) may be useful, and conventional antipsychotics or clozapine (C) may be required when atypical antipsychotics are not effective (second-line).

improvement than conventional antipsychotics (Fig. 2–55, first-line treatment); quetiapine and ziprasidone have so far documented better negative symptom improvement than placebo (Fig. 2–55, second-line treatment).

Use of Atypical Antipsychotics for Treating Hostility, Aggression, and Poor Impulse Control in Schizophrenia and Related Disorders

Patients with schizophrenia can obviously be hostile and aggressive, toward self, staff, family, and property. This may take the form of suicide attempts, self-mutilation, poor impulse control, drug abuse, verbal abuse, physical abuse, and/or threatening behavior and may not directly correlate with positive symptoms. It can be a particular problem in a forensic setting. Such problems are commonly a symptom dimension in many psychiatric disorders other than schizophrenia, including many childhood and adolescent disorders such as conduct disorder, oppositional defiant disorder, autism, mental retardation, and attention deficit hyperactivity disorder, as well as borderline personality disorder, bipolar disorders, and various types of organic disorders and brain damage, including head injury, stroke, and Alzheimer's disease (see Chapter 1 and Fig. 1–5). This dimension of psychopathology obvious cuts a wide swath across psychiatric disorders and is not necessarily associated with psychosis. Both conventional and atypical antipsychotics reduce such symptoms (Fig. 2–56), but there are far more studies of hostility and aggression in psychotic illnesses than in nonpsychotic illnesses.

Receptor Binding Properties of
Conventional Antipsychotics

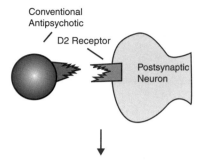

Tight, Long-Lasting Binding by
Conventional Antipsychotics

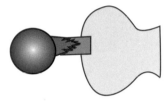

FIGURE 2–57. **Receptor binding properties of conventional antipsychotics.** Shown on the left is an icon for conventional antipsychotic drugs. Because of the biochemical properties of these drugs, their binding to postsynaptic D2 dopamine receptors is tight and long-lasting, as shown by the teeth on the binding site of the conventional antipsychotic. The D2 receptor on the right has grooves at which the teeth of the drug can bind tightly. *Tight, long-lasting binding by conventional antipsychotics:* Here the conventional antipsychotic is binding to the D2 postsynaptic receptor, with its teeth locking the drug into the receptor binding site to block it in a long-lasting manner.

Novel Theories About Dopamine 2 Receptors and Antipsychotic Mechanisms

Every known antipsychotic agent with efficacy for positive symptoms of psychosis has actions at D2 dopamine receptors. However, not all of the actions of effective antipsychotics at D2 receptors are the same. Indeed, some of the most interesting ideas about the newer antipsychotics are novel theories about the various ways that drugs can interact with these critical D2 receptors.

"Hit and Run" Actions at Dopamine Receptors: Possible Mechanism of Action of Atypical Antipsychotics

One current leading hypothesis states that antipsychotic actions require only transient blockade of D2 dopamine receptors in the mesolimbic dopamine pathway, but extrapyramidal side effects require long-lasting blockade of D2 receptors in the nigrostriatal pathway. Therefore, if an antipsychotic blocks D2 receptors by tight and long-lasting binding (Fig. 2–57), not only do antipsychotic effects result, but so do motor side effects. However, if an antipsychotic blocks D2 receptors and then rapidly dissociates from them ("hit and run" action; Fig. 2–58), it would have

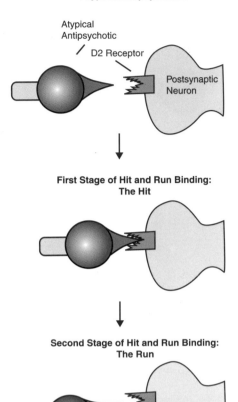

Receptor Binding Properties of Atypical Antipsychotics

FIGURE 2–58. **Receptor binding properties of atypical antipsychotics.** Shown on the left of this figure is the icon for atypical antipsychotic drugs. Because of their biochemical nature, the binding of atypical antipsychotics to postsynaptic D2 dopamine receptors on the right is loose, as shown by a smooth binding site for the atypical antipsychotic, which does not fit into the teeth of the receptor. *First stage of hit and run binding: The hit.* Here the atypical antipsychotic is binding to the D2 dopamine receptor. Note that it fits loosely into the D2 receptor without getting locked into the grooves of the receptor as do conventional antipsychotics. *Second stage of hit and run binding: The run.* Since an atypical antipsychotic fits loosely into the D2 receptor, it slips off easily after binding only briefly and then runs away. This is also called *rapid dissociation.*

atypical antipsychotic properties, namely reduction of psychosis without motor side effects. The improved tolerability of these atypical antipsychotics would thus be theoretically linked to reduced D2 receptor blockade in parts of the brain where side effects are mediated.

The hypothetical actions of a conventional antipsychotic over time (Fig. 2–59) are thus theoretically distinct from those of atypical antipsychotics (Fig. 2–60). When conventional antipsychotics block D2 receptors throughout the brain, they

Hypothetical Action of a Conventional
Antipsychotic Over Time

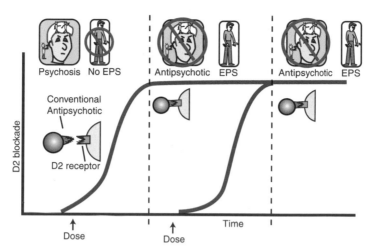

FIGURE 2–59. **Hypothetical action of a conventional antipsychotic over time.** This figure shows a curve of D2 receptor blockade after two doses of a conventional antipsychotic, as well as the concomitant clinical effects. *Prior to dosing* a schizophrenic patient with a conventional antipsychotic (far left), there is no D2 receptor blockade, and the schizophrenic patient has positive symptoms of psychosis such as delusions and hallucinations (indicated by the Martian speaking in the patient's ear and dancing in his head). Also, since there is no drug present, there will be no extrapyramidal motor side effects (EPS) (shown by a slash through the patient with parkinsonism). Following a dose of a conventional antipsychotic (middle), D2 receptors are blocked so tightly that they both cause antipsychotic actions and induce EPS. Following another dose of a conventional antipsychotic (far right), the D2 receptors stay persistently blocked, so that antipsychotic actions are always associated with EPS.

cannot produce antipsychotic actions without inducing motor side effects (Fig. 2–59). When atypical antipsychotics block D2 receptors, however, they stay around long enough to cause an antipsychotic action but not long enough to cause side effects (Fig. 2–60). According to this theory, reduced D2 receptor blockade is linked to the ability of an atypical antipsychotic drug to quickly dissociate from the receptor after blocking it and thus to produce antipsychotic actions without motor side effects. This is due to the nature of the biochemical properties of atypical antipsychotic drugs, which results in loose binding to the D2 receptor. Binding of an atypical antipsychotic is theoretically tight enough and long-lasting enough initially to block the receptor and cause antipsychotic actions (the hit, Fig. 2–58) but loose enough and short enough in duration to slip off the receptor prior to inducing motor side effects (the run, Fig. 2–58).

Support for the hit and run hypothesis of atypical antipsychotic action is based in part on evidence from positron emission tomography (PET) scans of patients taking antipsychotics, showing that when dopamine 2 binding in the striatum is high, even in the presence of high 5HT2A binding in the cortex, motor side effects still occur. Also, rapid dissociation from the dopamine 2 receptor in vitro is a good predictor of low extrapyramidal side effect potential in patients. Since rapid dissociation

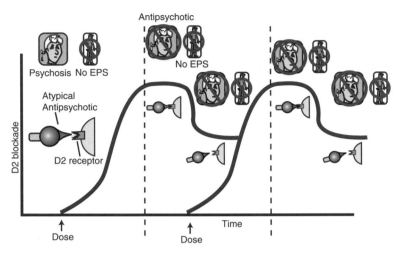

FIGURE 2–60. **Hypothetical action of an atypical antipsychotic over time.** This figure shows a curve of D2 receptor blockade after two doses of an atypical antipsychotic as well as the concomitant clinical effects. *Prior to dosing* a schizophrenic patient with an atypical antipsychotic (far left), there is no D2 receptor blockade, and the schizophrenic patient has positive symptoms of psychosis, just as in Fig. 2–59. Also, since there is no drug present, there will be no extrapyramidal motor side effects (EPS). *Following a dose of an atypical antipsychotic (middle),* D2 receptors are blocked initially, but then the drug slides off the receptor and they are no longer blocked. Theoretically, antipsychotic actions require only initial blockade of D2 receptors, whereas EPS require persistent blockade of D2 receptors. Since the nature of atypical antipsychotic binding is such that the drugs rapidly dissociate from D2 receptors after binding to them, these drugs can have antipsychotic actions without inducing EPS by hitting the D2 receptor hard enough to cause antipsychotic effects and then running before they cause EPS. Since this happens dose after dose (far right), there are persistent and long-lasting antipsychotic actions, but EPS do not develop over time.

means low potency, this also means that low-potency agents (i.e., those requiring higher milligram doses, such as clozapine and quetiapine) dissociate faster from the dopamine 2 receptor than do high-potency agents (i.e., those requiring lower milligram doses, such as risperidone), with intermediate-potency agents such as olanzapine in the middle. This roughly correlates with the abilities of these drugs to cause motor side effects within the group of atypical antipsychotics and also sets them all apart from the conventional antipsychotics.

One of the consequences of fast dissociation is that the drug is gone from the receptor until the next dose. This means that natural dopamine can bathe the receptor for a while before the next pulse of drug. Perhaps a bit of real dopamine in the nigrostriatal dopamine system is all that is needed to prevent motor side effects. If this happens while there is yet insufficient dopamine in the mesolimbic dopamine system to reactivate psychosis between doses, the drug has atypical antipsychotic clinical properties (Fig. 2–60).

Dopamine Stimulant

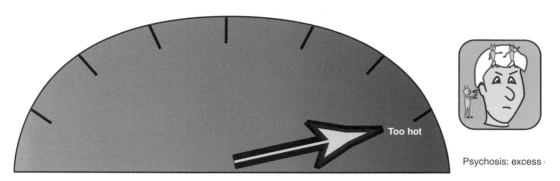

FIGURE 2–61. This action is too hot; excess of full agonist.

Conventional Antipsychotic

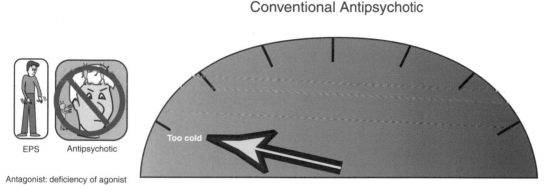

FIGURE 2–62. This action is too cold; powerful antagonist actions accompanied by deficiency of agonist action.

Dopamine System Stabilizers: The "Goldilocks" Antipsychotics

A new class of antipsychotics is emerging that interacts with D2 dopamine receptors in a novel manner. These new agents stabilize dopamine neurotransmission and may result in a binding to dopamine 2 receptors that is not too stimulating (Fig. 2–61), not too antagonizing (Fig. 2–62), but just right (Fig. 2–63).

What is dopamine system stabilization? It is a new concept for the action of antipsychotic drugs that do not induce motor side effects. The brain normally stabilizes dopamine neurotransmission by making sure that the dopamine output stimulating its receptors is sufficient but not excessive. Dopamine systems attain this state naturally by balancing the outputs of presynaptic and postsynaptic D2 receptors. For example, if dopamine output from the postsynaptic receptor is excessive, the presynaptic receptor just turns off further dopamine release, and the net output

Dopamine Stabilizer

Antipsychotic without EPS

Partial agonist: balance between agonist and antagonist actions

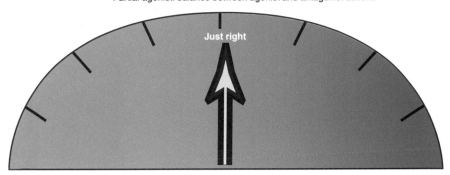

FIGURE 2–63. This action is just right; partial agonist as well as balance between agonist and antagonist actions.

from the system is diminished. In physiological states, dopamine systems would be stabilized, for example, when excessive dopamine activation needs to be reduced in one part of the brain while dopamine activity needs to continue normally in another part of the brain. This is possible because dopamine release gets turned off in a specific synapse when its concentrations become too high, but dopamine release continues elsewhere if its concentrations there are normal or low.

Presynaptic D2 receptors are responsible for regulating dopamine release. They are less sensitive to dopamine than are postsynaptic D2 receptors, so physiological neurotransmission continues until dopamine levels build up sufficiently to stimulate the presynaptic D2 receptors, thereby turning off further dopamine release.

Regional differences can exist within the brain for sensitivity of various pre- and postsynaptic D2 receptors to dopamine. Such differences can be due to changes in disease states that affect D2 receptors, drugs that affect D2 receptors, or physiological changes in the numbers of such receptors or the tightness with which these receptors are coupled to their second-messenger systems. The concept of dopamine system stabilization is to enhance or preserve dopaminergic neurotransmission where it is low, yet reduce dopaminergic neurotransmission where it is too high. In terms of treating psychosis, the goal is to reduce theoretically hyperactive dopamine neurons that mediate psychosis and at the same time to enhance theoretically underactive dopamine neurons that mediate negative and cognitive symptoms, while preserving physiological function in dopamine neurons that regulate motor movement and prolactin. This is supposed to all happen in the same brain at the same time.

How does a drug stabilize dopamine systems? Dopamine itself causes full receptor output from D2 receptors (Fig. 2–64A). Conventional antipsychotics are full antagonists and allow little or no output from D2 receptors (Fig. 2–64B). However,

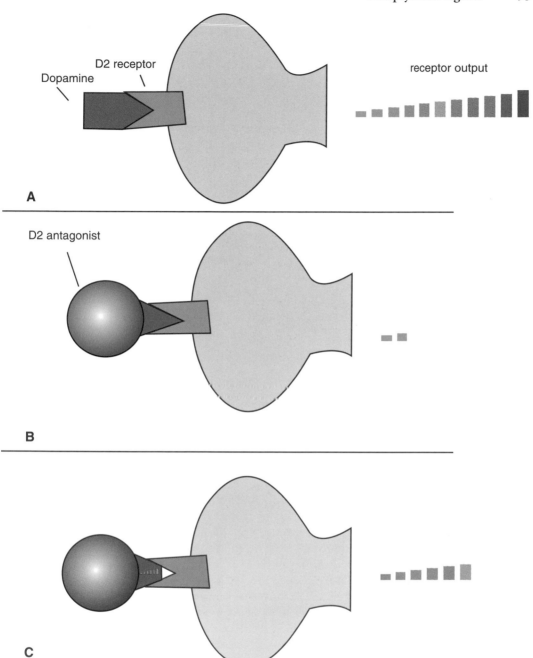

FIGURE 2–64. Dopamine itself is a full agonist and causes full receptor output (A). Conventional antipsychotics are full antagonists and allow little if any receptor output (B). Dopamine system stabilizers partially activate dopamine receptor output and cause a stabilizing balance between stimulation and blockade of dopamine receptors (C).

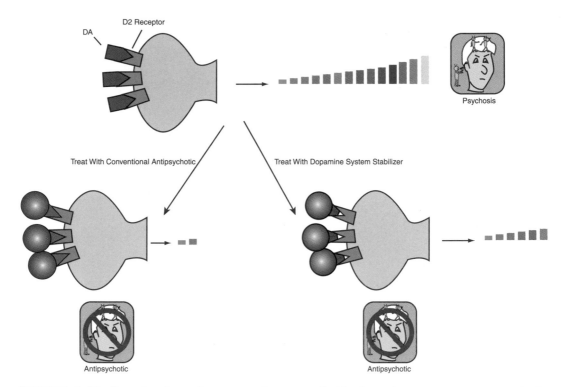

FIGURE 2–65. Excessive dopamine output from mesolimbic dopamine neurons causes psychosis. Both conventional antipsychotics and dopamine system stabilizers reduce this output. Although the reduction in dopamine output is not as robust for the dopamine system stabilizers as for the conventional antipsychotics, it is reduced sufficiently with enough stabilization to produce a comparable degree of antipsychotic action.

a dopamine system stabilizer achieves a balance between agonist and antagonist actions, resulting in an intermediate amount of output from D2 receptors (Fig. 2–64C). Dopamine system stabilizers are therefore far different from receptor antagonists, which always block the action of dopamine completely, thereby keeping physiological output from D2 receptors "silent". Dopamine system stabilizers are also very different from dopamine itself, a full agonist at D2 receptors, which creates maximum action and if the dose is high enough, even makes D2 receptors "scream". Dopamine system stabilizers, on the other hand, are like a pleasant conversation rather than either silence or shouting. Thus, when dopamine activity is silent, a dopamine system stabilizer increases dopamine output, but to a level not as "loud" as real dopamine (Fig. 2–64). In the presence of screaming maximum dopamine, dopamine system stabilizers reduce dopamine output to the dull roar of a pleasant conversation.

When dopamine is unable to stabilize its own neurotransmission in psychoses such as schizophrenia because of too much dopamine-induced D2 receptor output in mesolimbic dopamine pathways (Fig. 2–65), both a conventional antipsychotic and an atypical antipsychotic reduce excessive dopamine output there enough to produce antipsychotic actions (Fig. 2–65). However, only the dopamine

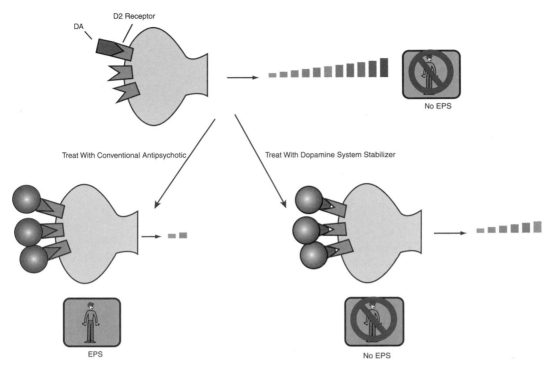

FIGURE 2 66. Dopaminergic tone in nigrostriatal neurons must be maintained for optimal motor functioning. Conventional antipsychotics reduce this tone so much that extrapyramidal motor side effects are produced. On the other hand, dopamine system stabilizers allow continuing dopaminergic tone in these neurons, so that motor side effects are not produced.

system stabilizer simultaneously allows sufficient output from nigrostriatal neurons so that motor tone is preserved, whereas conventional antipsychotics dampen nigrostriatal output so much that extrapyramidal side effects are the result (Fig. 2–66).

Another way to understand dopamine system stabilizers is to compare them with D2 receptor agonists and antagonists across a spectrum relating to their actions in psychosis. Thus, a full agonist dopamine stimulant is "too hot," causing or worsening psychosis (Fig. 2–61). A full antagonist is "too cold," yielding antipsychotic actions but at the cost of inducing extrapyramidal motor side effects (Fig. 2–62). In the middle, a dopamine system stabilizer could be "just right," with the ability to cause antipsychotic actions without inducing motor side effects (Fig. 2–63). Pharmacologically, this is known as *partial agonist action,* which means activation at low dopaminergic tone and inhibition at high dopaminergic tone, thus stabilizing dopamine output from either direction.

Molecularly, the exact mechanism of partial agonist binding to D2 receptors remains somewhat obscure, but it is hypothesized to exploit differences in D2 receptors pre- versus postsynaptically, in various brain regions, or in their affinities, distribution, density, and tightness of coupling to a physiological output. Clinically, the term "partial agonist" can be misinterpreted because "partial" can imply weak or incomplete. Dopamine system stabilizers, however, are not less effective than other types of antipsychotics. The prototypical member of this class, aripiprazole (also

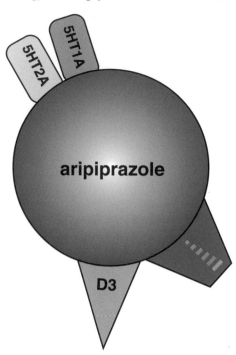

FIGURE 2–67. **Aripiprazole** pharmacologic icon, portraying a qualitative consensus of current thinking about binding properties of this drug. As for all atypical antipsychotics discussed in this chapter,
binding properties vary greatly with technique and species and from one laboratory to another; they
are constantly being revised and updated.

known as OPC-14597 or Abilitat), has been found in early clinical trials to reduce
psychosis as effectively as other antipsychotics without causing motor side effects
in schizophrenia. Aripiprazole also has serotonin 1A binding properties, which may
contribute to its clinical properties (Fig. 2–67).

Other agents in this class include (-)-3-(3-hydroxyphenyl)-N-n-propylpiperidone
(3-ppp or precamol), OSU-6162, DU-127090, and WAY135,452. These agents all
have preclinical profiles as dopamine system stabilizers, with partial agonist effects
pharmacologically that predict antipsychotic actions without motor side effects. The
trick is to find an agent that allows sufficient dopamine action in nigrostriatal pathways to prevent motor side effects from developing while reducing dopamine sufficiently in mesolimbic pathways to cause antipsychotic actions. Too little dopamine
system stabilization, and there would not be antipsychotic actions. Too much
dopamine system stabilization, and you would have a conventional antipsychotic.
Early clinical development of several dopamine system stabilizers is ongoing or
imminent, and testing of aripiprazole is in late stages. Dopamine system stabilization may also help to explain some of the atypical clinical actions of benzamide
antipsychotics such as sulpiride and amisulpride (Fig. 2–68). Amisulpride acts only
at D2 and D3 receptors and lacks significant serotonin 2A antagonist properties
common to many atypical antipsychotics, yet it may have somewhat atypical clinical properties, with lower extrapyramidal motor side effects yet demonstrable
antipsychotic therapeutic effects.

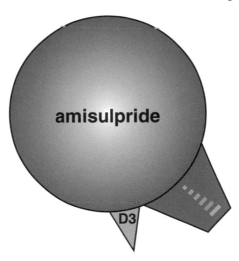

FIGURE 2–68. **Amisulpride** pharmacologic icon, portraying a qualitative consensus of current think-ing about binding properties of this drug. As for all atypical antipsychotics discussed in this chapter, binding properties vary greatly with technique and species and from one laboratory to another; they are constantly being revised and updated.

Atypical Antipsychotics as Mood Stabilizers for Bipolar Disorder

Classically, antipsychotics have always been distinguished from mood stabilizers in psychopharmacology. Thus, antipsychotics discussed in this chapter so far include both conventional antipsychotics and atypical antipsychotics; these agents are usu-ally emphasized as treatments for psychotic disorders, especially schizophrenia. On the other hand, the term "mood stabilizer" has generally implied lithium and cer-tain anticonvulsants that are emphasized for the stabilization of mood disorders, especially bipolar disorder. New observations are now making this conceptualiza-tion of antipsychotics as distinct from mood stabilizers obsolete, because atypical antipsychotics are now known to be effective in mania, not just psychotic mania but also in nonpsychotic, euphoric, rapid cycling, and mixed mania. Furthermore, so-called mood stabilizers such as lithium and various anticonvulsants are now known to boost the efficacy of atypical antipsychotics, not only in nonpsychotic mania but also in psychotic illnesses such as psychotic mania and treatment-resist-ant schizophrenia. This section will discuss the use of atypical antipsychotics as mood stabilizers for the treatment of bipolar disorder. Later, we will discuss the use of lithium and mood-stabilizing anticonvulsants as augmenting agents to boost the efficacy of antipsychotics in the treatment of schizophrenia and other psy-choses, especially those with inadequate treatment responses to antipsychotics alone.

Bipolar Disorder and a Brainstorm of Ions

Mania is an elevated, expansive, or irritable mood; hypomania is a less severe form of this (Fig. 2–69). Sometimes mania cycles quickly to depression and back to mania again; if this occurs with four distinct periods of abnormal mood within

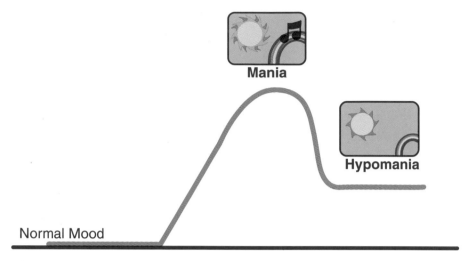

FIGURE 2–69. Mania is characterized by an elevated, expansive, or irritable mood. A less severe form of this is known as hypomania.

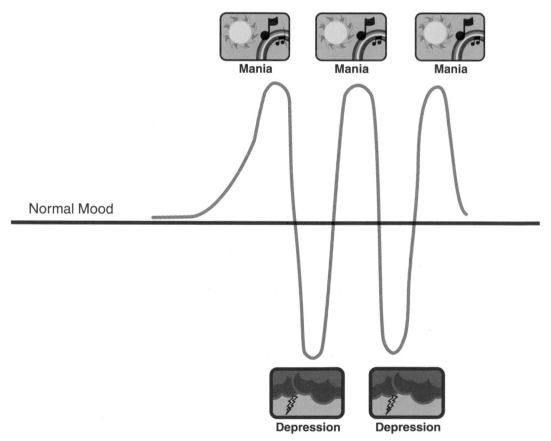

FIGURE 2–70. Mania can cycle quickly to depression and back to mania again. If this occurs with four distinct periods of abnormal mood within 1 year, it is called rapid cycling.

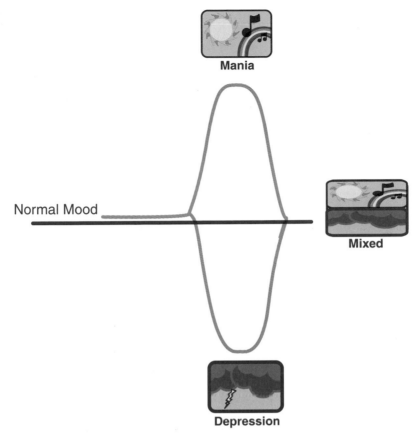

FIGURE 2–71. When features of mania and depression are present together, often associated with dysphoria or agitated depression, this is called a mixed state.

1 year, it is called rapid cycling (Fig. 2–70). The simultaneous presence of features of mania and depression, often associated with dysphoria or agitated depression, is called a mixed state (Fig. 2–71). Mania can also be associated with other clinical features, including drug and alcohol abuse, aggression, and psychosis (Fig. 2–72).

Although the pathophysiology of these abnormal unstable moods is not known, it may be linked to abnormal neuronal activity with increased ionic flow through ion channels in an electrical storm, which is analogous to ictal states such as seizure. Thus, some hypotheses suggest that increased ion flux specifically through voltage-gated ion channels (Fig. 2–73) may be associated with unstable mood states, especially mania (Fig. 2–74A and B). When dopamine is simultaneously released excessively, this causes psychotic mania (Fig. 2–75). Theoretically, mood stabilizers that normalize the flux of ions would reduce mania and prevent mood instability, whereas antipsychotics that block dopamine receptors would reduce psychosis, as explained below.

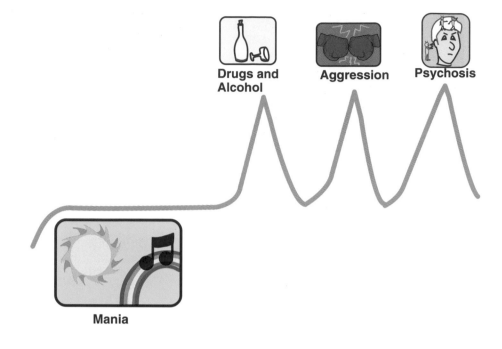

Normal Mood

FIGURE 2–72. Mania can be associated with other clinical features, including drug and alcohol abuse, aggression, and psychosis.

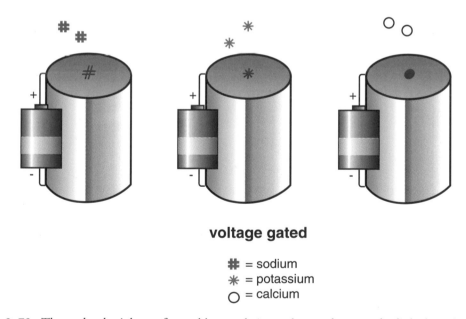

voltage gated

\# = sodium
✳ = potassium
○ = calcium

FIGURE 2–73. The pathophysiology of unstable moods is not known but may be linked to abnormal neuronal activity with increased ionic flow specifically through voltage-gated ion channels, which is analogous to ictal states such as seizures. Anticonvulsants are thought to reduce the flux of ions through voltage-gated ion channels, including those for sodium, potassium, and calcium ions.

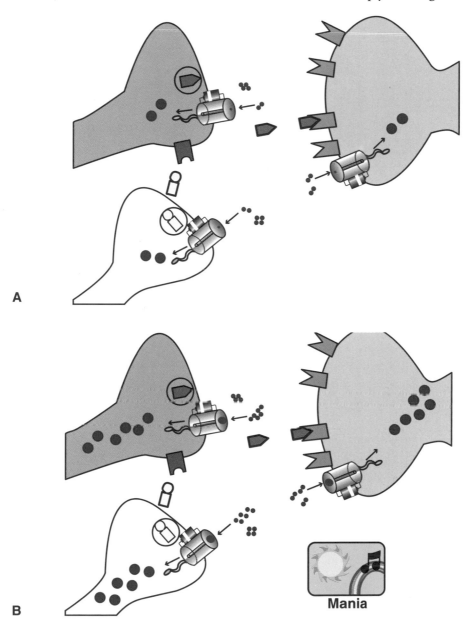

FIGURE 2–74. (A) Shown here is normal ion flux across neuronal membranes through voltage-gated ion channels. (B) Unstable mood states, particularly mania, are thought to be associated with increased ion flux across voltage-gated ion channels.

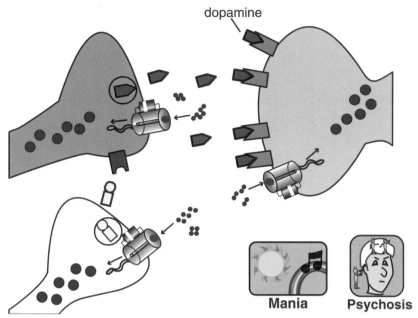

FIGURE 2–75. Psychosis associated with mania may be due to the same dopaminergic hyperactivity that causes psychosis in schizophrenia. Shown here is excessive dopamine release, leading to overstimulation of postsynaptic D2 receptors and consequently to delusions and hallucinations. When excessive release of dopamine occurs simultaneously with excessive ion flux through voltage-gated ion channels, psychotic mania results.

Mood-Stabilizing Drugs

Today, three classes of drugs act to reduce mania and stabilize mood: lithium, certain anticonvulsants, and certain atypical antipsychotics (Table 2–2).

Lithium, the classical mood stabilizer.   Bipolar disorder has classically been treated with lithium. Lithium is an ion whose mechanism of action is not certain, although it is hypothesized to interact with second messenger systems to result in a stabilization of ion flow in the neuron. Normally, signals are transduced from a neurotransmitter through its receptor to a second-messenger system, ultimately regulating ion channels, among many other things (Fig. 2–76A through G). It is possible that when these ion channels are opened excessively, mania and even seizures could result (Fig. 2–77). Lithium may reverse these actions by acting at G proteins that link

Table 2-2. *Three Classes of Mood Stabilizers*

Lithium
Anticonvulsants
divalproex
Atypical antipsychotics
olanzapine

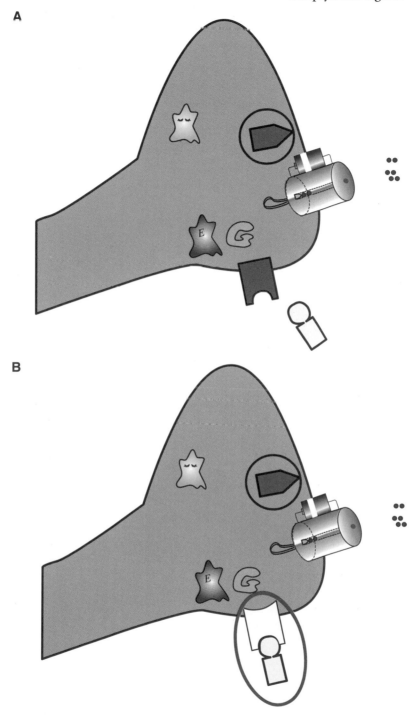

FIGURE 2–76. (A) Normal neuronal ion flow. Shown here is a second-messenger system, consisting of a neurotransmitter, in this case serotonin; a neurotransmitter receptor; a G protein; and an enzyme. Activation of the second-messenger system by the neurotransmitter results in the regulation of ion channels. (B) Serotonin binds to its receptor (red circle). *(Figure continues)*

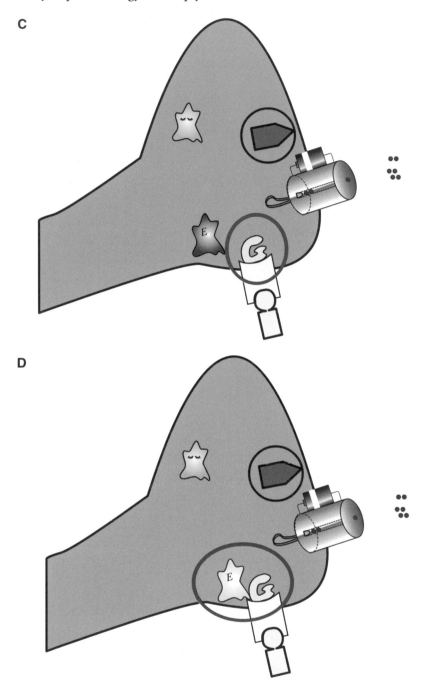

FIGURE 2–76 *(Continued)*. (C) Serotonin transforms the receptor so that it is capable of binding to a G protein (red circle). (D) The G protein is now able to bind to the enzyme capable of synthesizing the second messenger (red circle). *(Figure continues)*

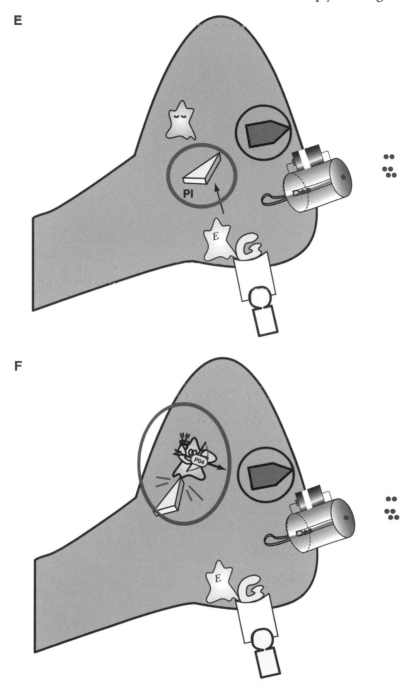

FIGURE 2–76 *(Continued).* (E) The second-messenger system phosphatidyl inositol (PI) is now activated, and the enzyme synthesizes this second messenger (red circle). (F) The second messenger activates an intracellular enzyme, readying it to phosphorylate the ion channel (red circle). *(Figure continues)*

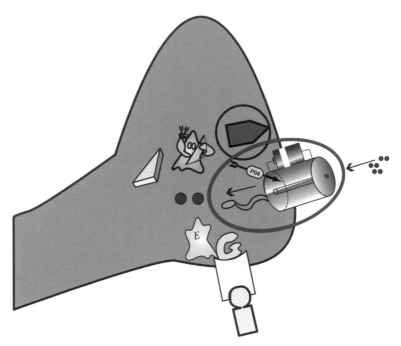

FIGURE 2–76 *(Continued).* (G) The intracellular enzyme phosphorylates the voltage-gated ion channel, opening it up and allowing for ion flux into the neuron (red circle).

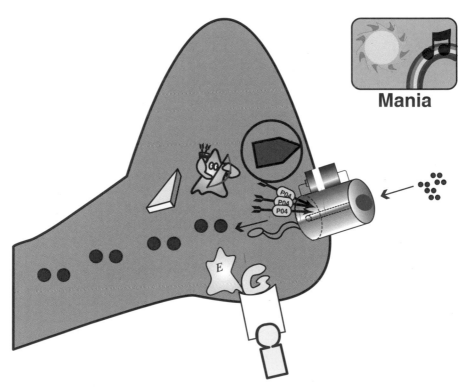

FIGURE 2–77. Shown here is excessive opening of voltage-gated ion channels, resulting in increased ionic flow into the neuron. This is thought to result in mania and even seizures.

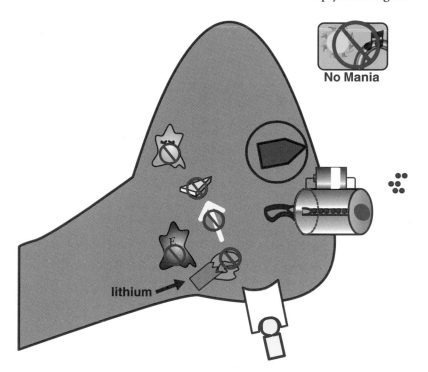

FIGURE 2 78. The mechanism of action of lithium is not well understood, but the ion is hypothesized to act by modifying second messenger systems. One possibility, depicted here, is that lithium alters G proteins and their ability to transduce signals inside the cell once the neurotransmitter receptor is occupied by the neurotransmitter. When this occurs, the neurotransmitter is not able to activate the second-messenger system to open the ion channel, and ion flux is reduced, normalizing mania and stabilizing moods.

neurotransmitter receptors to second-messenger systems (Fig. 2–78) or at enzymes that are part of the second-messenger system itself (Fig. 2–79) to bring about changes in ion flux through ion channels and thus normalize mania and stabilize moods. One leading idea is that lithium alters specifically the second messenger system phosphatidyl inositol and the associated enzyme inositol monophosphatase. Other actions of lithium result in changes in intracellular regulatory enzymes such as protein kinases and in gene expression (Figs. 2–78 and 2–79).

Lithium not only treats acute episodes of mania and hypomania (Fig. 2–80) but was the first psychotropic agent shown to prevent recurrent episodes of illness. Lithium may also be effective in treating and preventing episodes of depression in patients with bipolar disorder (Fig. 2–80). It is less effective for rapid cycling or mixed episodes. Overall, lithium is effective in only 40 to 50% of patients. Furthermore, many patients are unable to tolerate it because of numerous side effects, including gastrointestinal symptoms such as dyspepsia, nausea, vomiting, and diarrhea, as well as weight gain, hair loss, acne, tremor, sedation, decreased cognition, and incoordination. There are also long-term adverse effects on the thyroid and kidney. Lithium has a narrow therapeutic window, requiring monitoring of plasma drug levels.

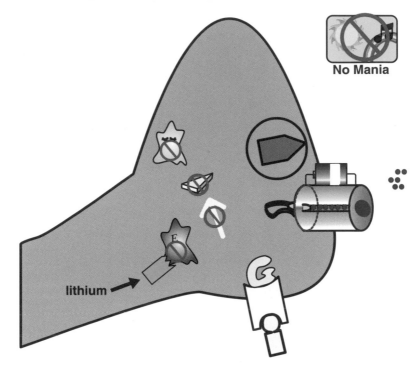

FIGURE 2–79. Lithium may also modify second-messenger systems by altering enzymes that inter-act with the second-messenger system, such as inositol monophosphatase or others. Again, this would prevent the second-messenger system from opening the ion channel, thereby reducing ion flux and normalizing mania.

Anticonvulsants as mood stabilizers.   Based on theories that mania may "kindle" fur-ther episodes of mania, a logical parallel with seizure disorders was drawn, since seizures can kindle more seizures. Thus, trials of several anticonvulsants, beginning with carbamazepine, have been conducted and are showing indications of efficacy for several anticonvulsants in treating the manic phase of bipolar disorder (Table 2–3). Valproic acid, formulated as divalproex, is the only anticonvulsant actually approved for this indication.

   The mechanism of action of anticonvulsants remains poorly characterized, whether in terms of their anticonvulsant effects or their anti-manic and mood-sta-bilizing effects. They may even have multiple mechanisms of action. The leading hypotheses for how anticonvulsants work are that they somehow reduce flux of ions through voltage-gated ion channels, including those for sodium, potassium, and calcium channels (Fig. 2–73). By interfering with sodium movements through volt-age-gated sodium channels, for example, several anticonvulsants cause use-depend-ent blockade of sodium inflow. That is, when the sodium channels are being "used" during neuronal activity, such as seizures or mania, anticonvulsants can prolong their inactivation, thus providing anticonvulsant and anti-manic mood-stabilizing actions.

   When another class of ion channels is inactivated, namely the ligand-gated ion channels (Fig. 2–81), changes of both excitatory and inhibitory neurotransmission

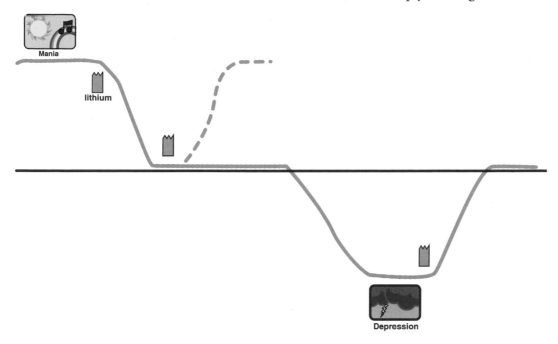

FIGURE 2–80. Lithium has documented efficacy in treating acute episodes of mania and hypomania. It also has been shown to prevent recurrent episodes of illness and may be effective in treating and preventing episodes of depression in patients with bipolar disorder as well.

result. Recall that glutamate is the universal excitatory neurotransmitter and gamma-aminobutyric acid (GABA) is the universal inhibitory neurotransmitter. In particular, several anticonvulsants appear to modulate the effects of the inhibitory neurotransmitter GABA by augmenting its synthesis, augmenting its release, inhibiting its breakdown, reducing its reuptake into GABA neurons, or augmenting its effects at GABA receptors (Fig. 2–81A). Some of these actions may be the mechanisms of anticonvulsant and anti-manic mood-stabilizing effects of these agents. Anticonvulsants that are also mood stabilizers may also interfere with neurotransmission by the excitatory neurotransmitter glutamate, in particular by reducing its release (Fig. 2–81B and C). Simply put, inhibitory neurotransmission with GABA may be enhanced and excitatory neurotransmission with glutamate may be reduced by anticonvulsant mood stabilizers.

Table 2–3. *Some anticonvulsants used to treat the manic phase of manic-depressive disorder*

Generic Name	Trade Name
Valproate/Divalproex	Depakene, Depakote, Depakote ER
Carbamazepine	Tegretol
Gabapentin	Neurontin
Topiramate	Topamax
Lamotrigine	Lamictal

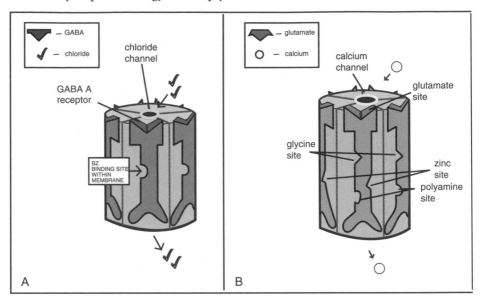

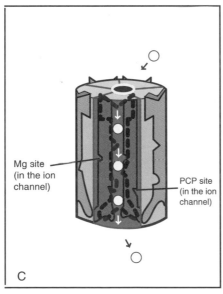

FIGURE 2–81. (A) Anticonvulsants such as benzodiazepines enhance the inhibitory actions of gamma-aminobutyric acid (GABA) by binding to ligand-gated ion channels associated with the GABA A receptor. They also appear to modulate the inhibitory effects of GABA by augmenting its synthesis, augmenting its release, inhibiting its breakdown, and reducing its reuptake into GABA neurons. (B&C). When the excitatory neurotransmitter glutamate binds to its receptor on the ligand-gated ion channel depicted here, it causes the calcium channel to open and the neuron to be excited for neurotransmission. Anticonvulsants that are also mood stabilizers may interfere with neurotransmission by glutamate, in particular by reducing its release.

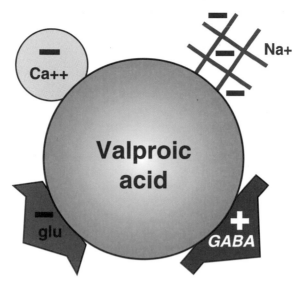

FIGURE 2–82. Shown here is an icon of the pharmacologic actions of **valproic acid.** By interfering with calcium channels and sodium channels, valproate is thought both to enhance the inhibitory actions of GABA and to reduce the excitatory actions of glutamate.

Other actions of anticonvulsant mood stabilizers include inhibition of the enzyme carbonic anhydrase, negative modulation of calcium channel activity, and actions on second-messenger systems, including inhibition of phosphokinase C. Beyond the second-messenger, there is the possibility that second-messenger systems may be affected, in analogy with what is hypothesized for lithium, leading ultimately not only to changes in ion flux through channels but also to changes in gene expression.

Valproic acid. Although its exact mechanism of action remains uncertain, valproic acid (also valproate sodium or valproate, often formulated as divalproex sodium) may inhibit sodium and/or calcium channel function and perhaps thereby boost GABA inhibitory action as well as reduce glutamate excitatory action (Fig. 2–82). Alterations of ion flux through voltage-gated ion channels may be either due to actions of valproic acid on enzymes that phosphorylate components of the channel (Fig. 2–83) or due to direct actions on the channel itself (Fig. 2–84). A unique and patented pharmaceutical formulation of valproic acid, called divalproex (Depakote and Depakote ER), reduces gastrointestinal side effects.

The Depakote (divalproex) form of valproic acid is approved for the acute phase of bipolar disorder. It is also commonly used for long-term maintenance to prevent relapses and recurrences, although its prophylactic effects have not been as well established as its effects on acute mania. Valproic acid is now frequently used as first-line treatment for bipolar disorders, as well as in combination with lithium for patients refractory to lithium monotherapy, and especially for patients with rapid cycling and mixed episodes (Fig. 2–85). Oral loading can lead to rapid stabilization, and plasma levels are monitored to keep drug levels within the therapeutic range. Valproic acid can also have unacceptable side effects, such as hair loss, weight

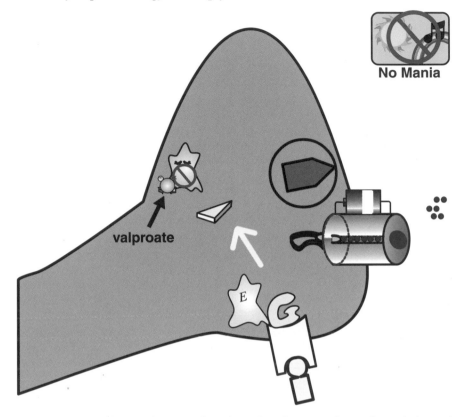

FIGURE 2–83. Valproic acid may alter ion flux through voltage-gated ion channels by acting on enzymes that regulate the phosphorylation of proteins that control the opening of ion channels.

gain, and sedation. Certain problems can limit valproic acid's usefulness in women of childbearing potential, including the fact that it can cause neural tube defects in the developing fetus. Menstrual disturbances, polycystic ovaries, hyperandrogenism, obesity, and insulin resistance as well as pancreatitis may also be associated with valproic acid therapy.

Carbamazepine.   Carbamazepine was actually the first anticonvulsant to be shown to be effective in the manic phase of bipolar disorder, but it has not been approved for this use by regulatory authorities such as the FDA. Its mechanism of action may be to enhance GABA function, perhaps in part by actions on sodium and/or potassium channels (Fig. 2–86). Because its efficacy is less well documented and its side effects can include sedation and hematological abnormalities, it is not as well accepted for first-line use in the treatment of mood disorders as either lithium or valproic acid.

Lamotrigine.   Lamotrigine is approved as an anticonvulsant but not as a mood stabilizer. It is postulated to inhibit sodium channels and to inhibit the release of

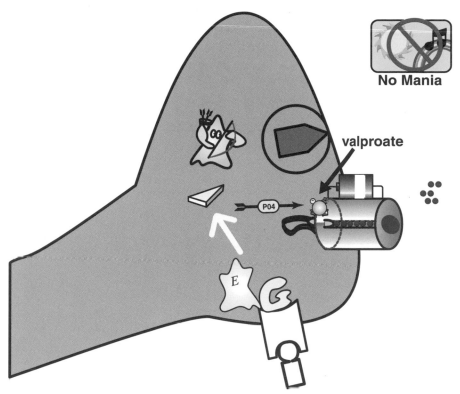

No Mania

valproate

FIGURE 2–84. Another possible explanation for how valproic acid alters ionic flow is that it binds directly to the channel itself, reducing its ability to conduct ions and thus relieving mania.

glutamate (Fig. 2–87). Numerous reports suggest that lamotrigine not only is able to stabilize bipolar manic and mixed episodes but also may be useful for the depressive episodes of this disorder. Further testing of lamotrigine's safety and efficacy in mood disorders is ongoing. This agent causes skin rashes, including a potentially dangerous skin reaction known as the Stevens-Johnson syndrome.

Gabapentin.   Gabapentin was synthesized as a GABA analogue but turned out not to directly modulate the GABA receptor. It may well interact at the GABA transporter and increase GABA levels (Fig. 2–88). It also decreases glutamate levels. It is approved as an anticonvulsant and was originally observed to improve mood and quality of life in seizure disorder patients. Numerous studies suggest efficacy in the manic phase of bipolar disorder, and further clinical evaluation as a mood stabilizer is ongoing. A gabapentin analogue called pregabalin is also undergoing clinical evaluation as an anticonvulsant and as a mood stabilizer.

Topiramate.   Topiramate is another compound that has been approved as an anticonvulsant and is in clinical testing as a mood stabilizer. Its mechanism of action appears to be enhancement of GABA function and reduction of glutamate function by interfering with both sodium and calcium channels. In addition, it is a

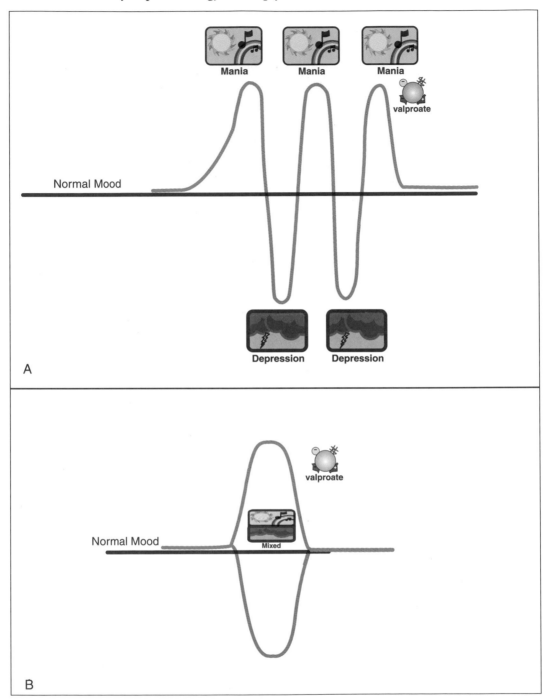

FIGURE 2–85. Valproic acid is often a first-line choice to treat patients with rapid cycling and mixed episodes.

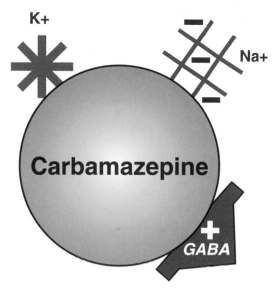

FIGURE 2–86. Shown here is an icon of **carbamazepine** pharmacologic actions. By interfering with sodium and potassium channels, carbamazepine is thought to enhance the inhibitory actions of GABA.

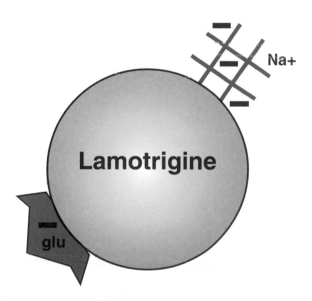

FIGURE 2–87. Shown here is an icon of **lamotrigine** pharmacologic actions. By interfering with sodium channels, lamotrigine is thought to reduce the excitatory actions of glutamate.

weak inhibitor of carbonic anhydrase (Fig. 2–89). Topiramate's mood-stabilizing actions may occur at lower doses than its anticonvulsant actions. This compound also has the interesting side effect of weight loss in some patients, a unique effect among mood stabilizers, which generally cause weight gain.

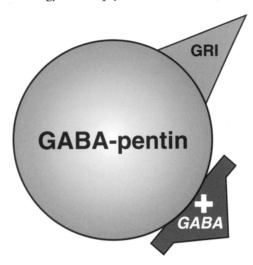

FIGURE 2–88. Shown here is an icon of **gabapentin** pharmacologic actions. Gabapentin is thought to act by enhancing GABA action, perhaps in part by inhibiting the reuptake of GABA into GABA terminals (shown as GRI [for GABA reuptake inhibition]) by blocking the GABA transporter. This enhances the inhibitory actions of GABA.

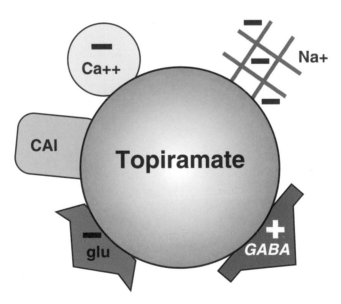

FIGURE 2–89. Shown here is an icon of **topiramate** pharmacologic actions. By interfering with calcium channels and sodium channels, topiramate is thought both to enhance the inhibitory actions of GABA and to reduce the excitatory actions of glutamate. Topiramate is also a carbonic anhydrase inhibitor (CAI), which has independent anticonvulsant actions.

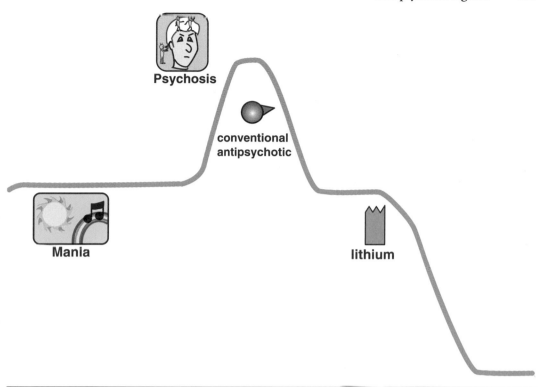

FIGURE 2–90. Psychosis associated with mania had long been treated with conventional antipsychotics as adjuncts to lithium or valproic acid, which are used to treat the mania itself.

Benzodiazepines.   Benzodiazepines, especially intravenous diazepam and oral clonazepam, have anticonvulsant actions. They are also sedating. Both of these actions have led to the use of benzodiazepines for the treatment of mood disorders, especially as an adjunctive treatment for agitation and psychotic behavior during the phase of acute mania. The mechanism of action of benzodiazepines is to enhance inhibitory neurotransmission at ligand-gated ion channels associated with the A receptor of GABA (Fig. 2–81A).

Conventional antipsychotics.   Classical neuroleptics (conventional antipsychotics) have long played a role in the treatment of agitation and psychosis associated with mania when given concomitantly with lithium or valproic acid, which were used to treat the mania itself (Fig. 2–90). However, this adjunctive use of conventional antipsychotics was associated with motor side effects and ultimately with tardive dyskinesia (Fig. 2–91). In the era prior to the advent of atypical antipsychotics, conventional antipsychotics thus had merely an adjunctive role in the treatment of bipolar disorders. This was not only because the actual anti-manic efficacy of conventional antipsychotics in nonpsychotic mania was poorly documented but also because it was not practical nor often ethical to maintain bipolar patients on such agents to prevent relapse in view of the unacceptable risk of tardive dyskinesia. Thus, conventional antipsychotics were reserved for short-term use in the treatment

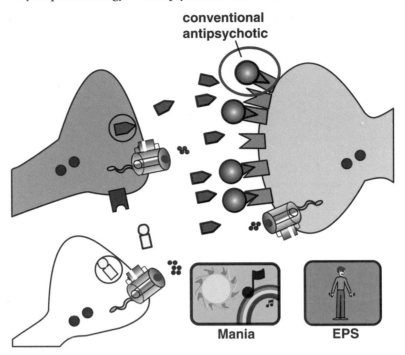

conventional antipsychotic

Mania   **EPS**

FIGURE 2–91. The blockade of dopamine D2 receptors by conventional antipsychotics reduces the psychosis associated with mania but does not affect the ion flow and thus does not reduce mania itself. Furthermore, the use of conventional antipsychotics is associated with motor side effects and ultimately with tardive dyskinesia. Thus, conventional antipsychotics are used only as adjunctive medications in the treatment of bipolar disorders, specifically for short-term treatment of acute episodes of mania, especially psychosis and aggression in hospitalized patients, or for treatment-resistant bipolar cases.

of acute episodes of mania, especially psychosis and aggression in hospitalized patients, or for treatment-resistant bipolar cases.

Atypical antipsychotics. More recently, the atypical antipsychotics have replaced older, conventional antipsychotics in their role as adjuncts to lithium or valproic acid in treating agitation and psychoses associated with mania (Fig. 2–92). This originally was mainly due to their improved tolerability and comparable or better antipsychotic efficacy of the newer agents, presumably resulting from their concomitant ability to block serotonin 2A receptors and thus reduce motor side effects (Fig. 2–93).

However, recent clinical experience with the atypical antipsychotics has led to observations that not only is there little or no risk of tardive dyskinesia with their long-term use, but also that they have surprising efficacy for mood symptoms in a number of disorders, ranging from improving depressed mood in schizophrenia, schizoaffective disorder, psychotic depression, and treatment-resistant depression. Large-scale studies have even proved that atypical antipsychotics are effective in nonpsychotic mania (Fig. 2–94) as well as in psychotic mania (Fig. 2–95) as monotherapies. Mixed cases, rapid cycling cases, and cases previously resistant to

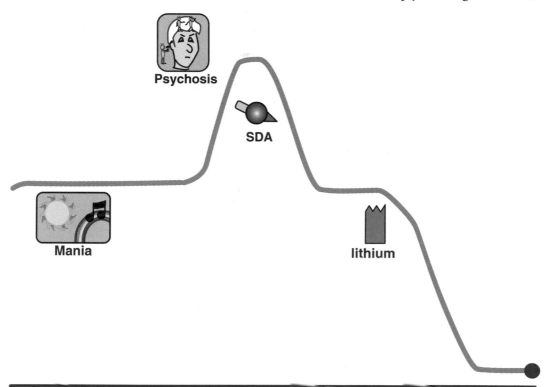

Psychosis

SDA

Mania

lithium

FIGURE 2–92. Recently, atypical antipsychotics have replaced older conventional antipsychotics as adjuncts to lithium or valproic acid in treating agitation and psychosis associated with mania.

lithium and anticonvulsants are also improved by atypical antipsychotics, and now one of these, olanzapine, has actually been approved as a monotherapy for treatment of acute mania. Studies of several other atypical antipsychotics in acute mania are also in progress, as are long-term studies of relapse prevention. Presumably, some property of the atypical antipsychotics may serve to reduce the abnormal ion flux in mania (Fig. 2–96), as well as the excessive dopamine in psychosis (Fig. 2–93).

Bipolar combinations. Combination treatment with two or more psychotropic medications is the rule rather than the exception for the treatment of bipolar disorders (bipolar combos in Fig. 2–97). First-line treatment is now with either lithium, valproic acid, or olanzapine. When patients fail to stabilize in the acute manic phase with one of these first-line treatments, various combinations of these agents are used as second-line treatments. Third-line treatments are various combinations with several other anticonvulsant mood stabilizers (such as carbamazepine, lamotrigine, gabapentin, or topiramate) or atypical antipsychotic mood stabilizers (such as risperidone, quetiapine, clozapine, or ziprasidone).

If lithium, anticonvulsant, or atypical antipsychotic combination therapies are used, a benzodiazepine or a conventional antipsychotic may need to be added, especially for the most disturbed patients (Fig. 2–97). That is, sedating benzodiazepines can be used for lesser degrees of agitation (benzo assault weapon in Fig. 2–97), but

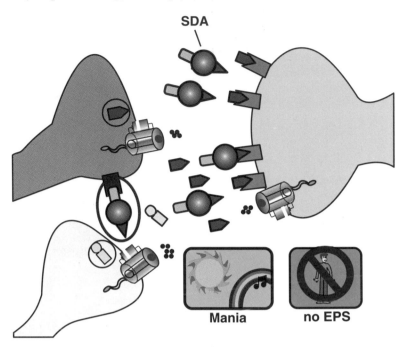

FIGURE 2–93. The use of atypical antipsychotics instead of conventional antipsychotics as adjuncts to lithium or valproic acid was originally mainly due to their improved tolerability and comparable or better antipsychotic efficacy, presumably because of their concomitant ability to block serotonin 2A receptors (red circle) and thus reduce motor side effects.

neuroleptic antipsychotics may be necessary for the most disturbed and out-of-control patients (nuclear weapon in Figure 2–97). Such drugs should be restricted to the acute phase and administered intermittently if possible.

Recommendations for maintenance treatment of bipolar disorder are undergoing rapid changes. In the recent past, lithium was the hallmark of maintenance treatment, often with antidepressant co-therapy for patients prone to depression as well as mania and not adequately controlled with lithium alone. Now, however, several new therapeutic principles are guiding the treatment of bipolar disorders in the maintenance phase.

First, anticonvulsants, particularly valproic acid, and atypical antipsychotics, especially olanzapine, are now considered excellent first-line choices as well as lithium, although lithium is the only agent approved for such use. Second, combinations of all three classes of mood stabilizers are recommended when monotherapies fail to prevent relapses. Third, antidepressant treatments are not benign in this condition. Although many bipolar patients were classically maintained on both lithium and an antidepressant, it is now recognized that antidepressants frequently decompensate bipolar patients, causing not only overt mania or hypomania but also the much more difficult to recognize and treat problems of mixed mania and rapid cycling. The trend today is to use antidepressants sparingly and if necessary, only in the presence of robust mood stabilization with one or more of the three classes of mood stabilizers. In fact, lithium, anticonvulsants, and atypical antipsychotics

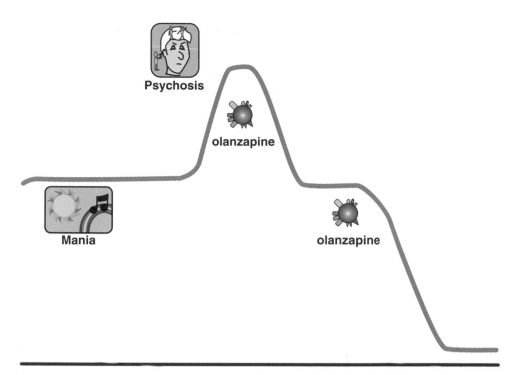

FIGURE 2–94. Large-scale studies have proved that atypical antipsychotics are effective as monotherapies in treating not only the psychotic symptoms but also the manic symptoms of psychotic mania.

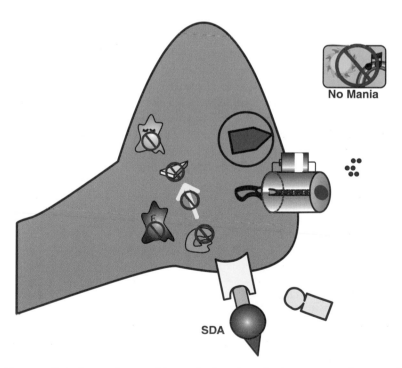

FIGURE 2–95. Recent clinical experience with atypical antipsychotics suggests that in addition to their antipsychotic effects and lack of motor side effects, they may have efficacy in treating mood symptoms in a number of disorders. Large-scale studies have even proved that atypical antipsychotics are effective as monotherapies in nonpsychotic mania.

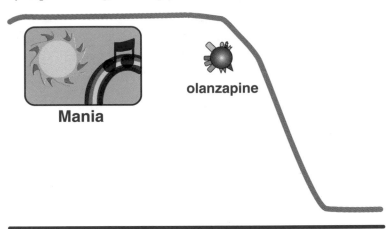

Mania   olanzapine

FIGURE 2–96. Presumably, some property of the atypical antipsychotics may serve to reduce the abnormal ion flux in mania. Mood-stabilizing properties of atypical antipsychotics may be related to their serotonin 2A–dopamine 2 receptor antagonism, or these drugs may alter the permeability of ion channels to close them.

may all be useful for the depressed and mixed manic–depressed phases of bipolar illness, reducing or perhaps eliminating the need for potentially destabilizing antidepressants in bipolar patients. Thus, antidepressants are now relegated to third-line use in bipolar disorder, behind lithium, anticonvulsant mood stabilizers, and atypical antipsychotics. This is an antidepressant-sparing strategy for the treatment of bipolar disorder.

Other combination maintenance treatments for bipolar disorder can include two or more mood stabilizers, with or without an atypical antipsychotic; a mood stabilizer and/or atypical antipsychotic with a benzodiazepine; a mood stabilizer with thyroid hormone; or even a mood stabilizer and/or atypical antipsychotic with an antidepressant (Fig. 2–97).

FIGURE 2–97. Combination treatments for bipolar disorder **(bipolar combos).** Combination drug treatment is the rule rather than the exception for patients with bipolar disorders. It is best to attempt monotherapy, however, with first-line lithium or valproic acid; with first- or second-line atypical antipsychotics; or with third-line anticonvulsant mood stabilizers. A very common situation in acute treatment of the manic phase of bipolar disorder is the use of both a mood stabilizer and an atypical antipsychotic (atypical combo). Agitated patients may require intermittent doses of sedating benzodiazepines (benzo assault weapon), whereas patients out of control may require intermittent doses of tranquilizing neuroleptics (neuroleptic nuclear weapon). For maintenance treatment, patients often require combinations of two mood stabilizers (mood stabilizer combo), or a mood stabilizer with an atypical antipsychotic (atypical combo). For patients who have depressive episodes despite mood stabilizer or atypical combos, antidepressants may be required (antidepressant combo). However, antidepressants may also decompensate patients into overt mania, rapid cycling states, or mixed states of mania and depression. Thus, antidepressant combos are used cautiously.

Bipolar Combos

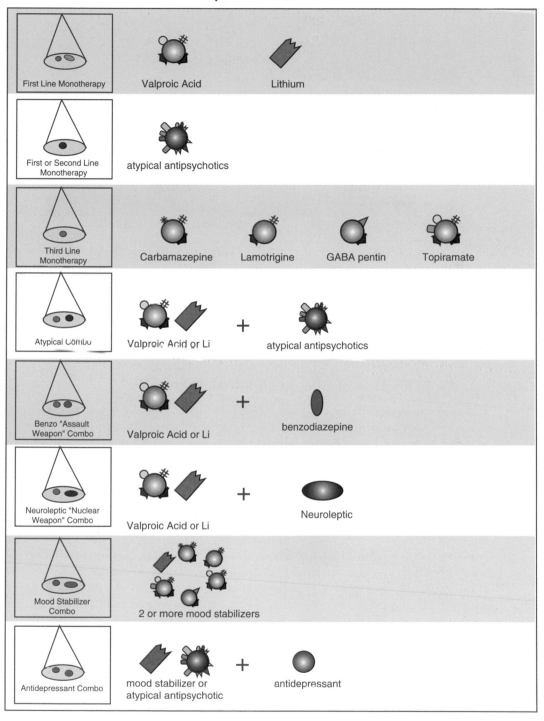

First Line Monotherapy	Valproic Acid	Lithium
First or Second Line Monotherapy	atypical antipsychotics	
Third Line Monotherapy	Carbamazepine Lamotrigine GABA pentin Topiramate	
Atypical Combo	Valproic Acid or Li + atypical antipsychotics	
Benzo "Assault Weapon" Combo	Valproic Acid or Li + benzodiazepine	
Neuroleptic "Nuclear Weapon" Combo	Valproic Acid or Li + Neuroleptic	
Mood Stabilizer Combo	2 or more mood stabilizers	
Antidepressant Combo	mood stabilizer or atypical antipsychotic + antidepressant	

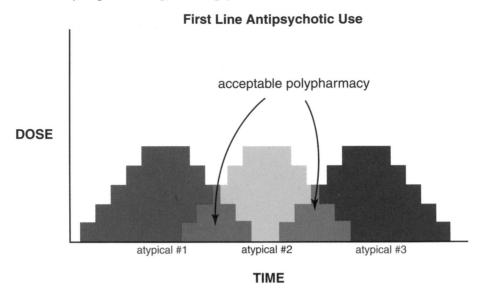

FIGURE 2–98. When switching from one atypical antipsychotic to another, it is frequently prudent to "cross-titrate," that is, to build down the dose of the first drug while building up the dose of the other. This leads to transient administration of two drugs, but is justified in order to reduce side effects and the risk of rebound symptoms and to accelerate the administration of the second drug.

Combining Drugs for Treatment-Resistant Schizophrenia

Schizophrenic patients usually respond to treatment with any single antipsychotic drug, whether conventional or atypical, with improvement of their positive symptoms of at least 30 or 40% on standardized rating scales after a month or two of treatment. However, if a treatment effect of this order of magnitude is not observed after an adequate trial with the first antipsychotic agent (usually an atypical antipsychotic agent, according to current treatment guidelines), most clinicians switch to another atypical antipsychotic drug. When switching from one atypical antipsychotic to another, it is frequently prudent to "cross-titrate," that is, to build down the dose of the first drug while building up the dose of the other (Fig. 2–98). This leads to transient administration of two drugs, but it is justified in order to reduce side effects and the risks of rebound symptoms as well as to accelerate the administration of the second drug. However, it is also possible to get trapped in cross-titration (Fig. 2–99). That is, when switching, the patient may improve in the middle of cross-titration, and the clinician may decide to continue both drugs rather than to complete the switch. This type of polypharmacy is not justified because current treatment guidelines (e.g., those from the American Psychiatric Association) recommend that only after several failures with sequential monotherapies, including consideration of clozapine, and conventional antipsychotic monotherapy, should long-term polypharmacy with two antipsychotics be given.

Conventional antipsychotics may occasionally be added to atypical antipsychotics to "lead in" the initiation of atypical antipsychotic administration for the treatment of positive symptoms when the more rapid onset of action of the conventional

Getting Trapped in Cross-Titration

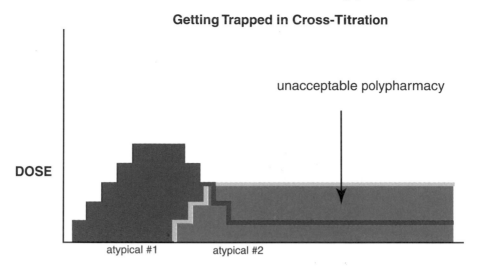

FIGURE 2–99. Getting caught in cross-titration. When switching from one atypical antipsychotic to another, the patient may improve in the middle of cross-titration. The polypharmacy that results if cross-titration is stopped and the patient continues both drugs indefinitely without a monotherapy trial of the second drug is not currently justified.

antipsychotics is necessary, and it then can be phased out while the atypical antipsychotics are phased in for maintenance in a less acute situation (Fig. 2–100). Conventional antipsychotics may also be useful to periodically "top up" patients on atypical antipsychotic maintenance treatment who are experiencing bouts of aggressiveness; in this situation they allow for more rapid and more robust relief of symptoms than an additional dose of the maintenance atypical antipsychotic (Fig. 2–100).

With four atypical antipsychotics, clozapine, and several conventional antipsychotics, one might expect that if one follows treatment guidelines, the odds of using long-term maintenance polypharmacy might be relatively low and something that might be reserved as a last resort and for the sickest of the sick. However, audits of antipsychotic use in clinical practice suggest that up to a fourth of outpatients and up to half of inpatients take two antipsychotic drugs for long-term maintenance treatment. Is this a viable therapeutic option for treatment-resistant patients or a dirty little secret of irrational drug use? Whatever it is, the use of two antipsychotics seems to be one of the most practiced and least investigated phenomena in clinical psychopharmacology. It may occasionally be useful to combine two agents when no single agent is effective. On the other hand, it has not proved useful to combine two antipsychotics to get supra-additive antipsychotic effects, such as "wellness" or "awakenings." Clinicians must remember that although *depressed* patients frequently recover, *schizophrenic* patients rarely achieve wellness, no matter what drug or drug combination is given. Thus, current treatment guidelines suggest that maintenance of patients on two antipsychotics or even very high doses of atypical antipsychotics should be done sparingly and perhaps only "when all else fails" (Fig. 2–101) and then continued only when clearly demonstrated to be beneficial.

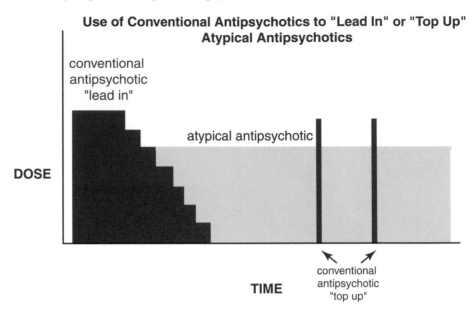

FIGURE 2–100. Use of conventional antipsychotics to "lead in" or "top up" atypical antipsychotics. One of the most important and justified uses of antipsychotic polypharmacy is to lead in to treatment with a conventional antipsychotic when an unmedicated patient is acutely psychotic, combative, or out of control. Such patients may also require periodic top-up for bouts of aggressiveness, allowing for more rapid and robust relief of symptoms than would be provided by an additional dose of the maintenance atypical antipsychotic.

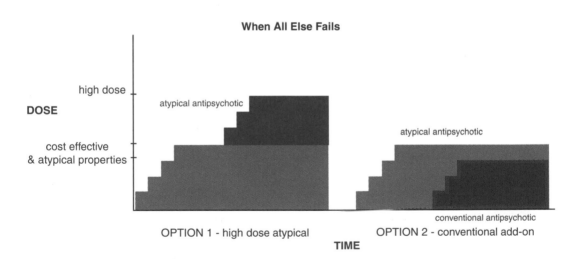

FIGURE 2–101. When all else fails, that is, if all of the atypical antipsychotics show insufficient efficacy, it may be necessary to use high doses. This is quite costly and leads to loss of the "atypical" therapeutic advantages of such drugs. Another option is to give a second antipsychotic from the conventional class to augment an inadequately efficacious atypical antipsychotic.

Antipsychotic polypharmacy, although frequently used in clinical practice, has very little controlled clinical trial data to support its use. In addition, it is very expensive to use two atypical antipsychotics together. Other possibilities rapidly gaining acceptance, including some well-designed clinical trials, are the augmentation of an atypical antipsychotic with a mood stabilizer, especially divalproex, with other anticonvulsants, or occasionally with lithium in order to augment inadequate treatment responses to an atypical antipsychotic in schizophrenia.

Other Antipsychotics

Loxapine is another serotonin-dopamine antagonist (SDA) with a structural formula related to that of clozapine (Figure 2–36) but unique pharmacological properties (Fig. 2–102). As usually dosed, it has an entirely conventional antipsychotic profile, including extrapyramidal motor side effects (EPS) and elevations in prolactin. There are hints, however, that it may be somewhat "atypical" at much lower than usually administered doses, and this is confirmed by human PET scans. It is one of the few agents available for intramuscular administration and usually causes no weight gain or even weight loss. A principal metabolite has noradrenergic reuptake blocking properties, suggesting possible antidepressant actions.

Zotepine, an SDA available in several European countries and Japan, has a chemical structure related to that of clozapine (Fig. 2–36) but with distinguishing pharmacologic (Fig. 2–103) and clinical properties. Although an SDA, some EPS have nevertheless been observed, as have prolactin elevations. As with clozapine, there is an increased risk of seizures, especially at high doses, as well as weight gain and sedation. However, there is no clear evidence yet that zotepine is as effective as clozapine for patients who fail to respond to conventional antipsychotics. It is interesting however, that zotepine inhibits norepinephrine reuptake, suggesting potential antidepressant actions. More clinical research is in progress to determine whether zotepine is superior to conventional antipsychotics or to atypical antipsychotics for the treatment of positive symptoms or negative symptoms.

Perospirone is a relatively new atypical antipsychotic that has been introduced into the Japanese market. This agent is a serotonin 2A–dopamine 2 antagonist like all the other atypical antipsychotics and has clinical signs of antipsychotic efficacy without a significant propensity to induce extrapyramidal motor side effects, as would be predicted from its pharmacology (Fig. 2–104).

Future Antipsychotics

Innovation in the area of schizophrenia is one of the most active areas in research in psychopharmacology. Although this is a most exciting topic, it may not be of interest to every reader, and especially not to the beginner nor to the generalist. For these readers, you may wish to skip to the end of the chapter, and to the summary.

Novel Serotonergic and Dopaminergic Mechanisms

Iloperidone is a compound in clinical development with SDA properties, but it has even more potent alpha 1 antagonist properties. It may have the possibility of being

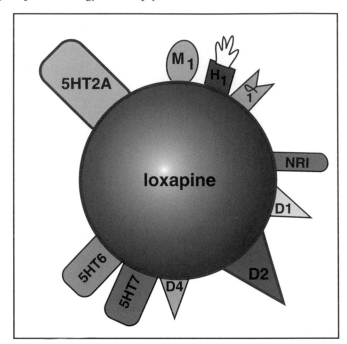

FIGURE 2–102. **Loxapine** pharmacologic icon, portraying a qualitative consensus of current think-ing about binding properties of this drug. As for all atypical antipsychotics discussed in this chapter, binding properties vary greatly with technique and species and from one laboratory to another; they are constantly being revised and updated.

developed into a much needed long-lasting depot formulation, none of which exist for any current atypical antipsychotic.

Mazapertine is a D2 antagonist, but rather than 5HT2A antagonist properties it has 5HT1A agonist actions. *Nemonapride* is a D2 (D3, D4) antagonist and 5HT1A agonist as well. MDL-100,907, a selective 5HT2A antagonist, was recently dropped from clinical development, as was the 5HT2A/2C antagonist ritanserin in prior years, both for lack of robust efficacy in schizophrenia. However, there remains some interest in some other nonspecific 5HT2A/2C antagonists such as SR 46349 and also in some 5HT2C selective agonists and antagonists. There are even novel and selective 5HT6 and 5HT7 antagonists also in development.

On the dopamine side of the equation, several D4 antagonists have been tested in schizophrenia, with generally disappointing results, although some trials are con-tinuing. Such compounds, some more selective for D4 receptors than others, include YM-43611, nemonapride, fananserin, L-745,870, PNU-101,387G, NGD-94-4, LU-111,995 among others. Several selective D3 antagonists are being developed because most known D2 antagonists also block D3 receptors. It is theoretically pos-sible that pure D3 antagonists, which increase psychomotor behavior in rodents, might activate such behaviors in schizophrenia and thus reduce negative symptoms. Other compounds in testing for schizophrenia include D1-like selective antagonists.

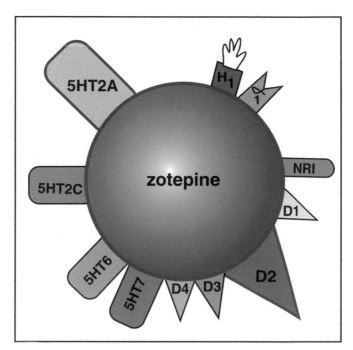

FIGURE 2–103. Zotepine pharmacologic icon, portraying a qualitative consensus of current thinking about the binding properties of this drug. As for all atypical antipsychotics discussed in this chapter, binding properties vary greatly with technique and species and from one laboratory to another; they are constantly being revised and updated.

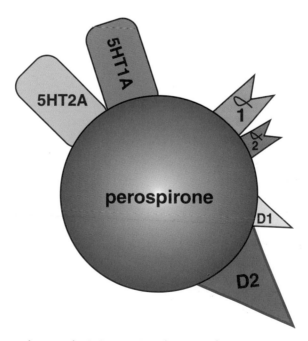

FIGURE 2–104. Perospirone pharmacologic icon, portraying a qualitative consensus of current thinking about the binding properties of this drug. As for all atypical antipsychotics discussed in this chapter, binding properties vary greatly with technique and species and from one laboratory to another; they are constantly being revised and updated.

Novel Neurotransmitter Mechanisms Other Than Serotonin and Dopamine for Therapeutic Strategies in Schizophrenia

Sigma antagonists. The physiological functions of the sigma receptor remain poorly characterized; thus, these receptors remain in many ways the "sigma enigma." Originally categorized as one of the opiate receptors, it is now associated with the actions of the psychotomimetic agent phencyclidine (PCP) and the activity of the NMDA subtype of glutamate receptors. Theoretically, a sigma antagonist could block any PCP-like actions occurring in schizophrenia. Although early testing of the sigma antagonist BMY-14,802 in schizophrenia was not impressive, other antagonists with greater selectivity have been developed and have entered testing. One, SR31742A, has not had robust clinical results in schizophrenia. A combined sigma/5HT1A agonist/5HT reuptake inhibitor OPC14523 is being tested in depression.

Cannabinoid antagonists. An antagonist to cannabinoid 1 (CB1) receptors, SR141716A, reduces the activity of mesolimbic dopamine neurons in animal models and blocks cannabinoid intoxication in humans. These results suggest possible antipsychotic actions in schizophrenia, but in early clinical testing in schizophrenic patients it has not shown robust efficacy.

Neurotensin antagonists. Neurotensin is a peptide neurotransmitter, which is co-localized with dopamine in the mesolimbic dopamine pathway but is much lower in concentration in nigrostriatal and mesocortical dopaminergic pathways. A nonpeptide antagonist SR-142948 is in clinical testing in schizophrenia as a theoretical agent that could reduce positive symptoms without producing EPS by exploiting differential actions on the mesolimbic rather than nigrostriatal dopamine systems. However, early clinical results of this agent are also not encouraging.

Cholecystokinin. Cholecystokinin (CCK) is also co-localized with dopaminergic neurons and has two receptor subtypes, CCK-A being predominantly outside and CCK-B within the central nervous system. Studies of CCK agonists and antagonists to date have not given clear clues as to their potential for therapeutic actions in schizophrenia.

Substance P and the neurokinins. Antagonists to all three neurokinin receptors (NK-1, NK-2, and NK-3) are now in clinical testing for a variety of indications, predominantly depression. Several are being tested in schizophrenia as well. Early clinical results with an NK-3 antagonist are intriguing.

Alpha-7-nicotinic cholinergic agonists. Although the role of therapeutics for cognition will be more extensively discussed in connection with cognitive enhancers, it is appropriate to consider the role of cognitive enhancers in schizophrenia as well, for this, too, is a disorder characterized in part by cognitive dysfunction. Furthermore, cholinergic deficiency may not be associated only with Alzheimer's disease, since the alpha-7-nicotinic cholinergic receptor has been implicated in the familial transmission of sensory gating deficits in families with schizophrenia. Deficits in activity at this receptor could theoretically predispose patients to problems with learning efficiency and accuracy and underlie delusional thinking and social dysfunction. In addition, heavy smoking in many schizophrenics (about two-thirds of a North American population of schizophrenics are smokers, as compared with about one-fourth of nonschizophrenics) is consistent with the high concentration of nicotine necessary to activate the receptor and with the receptor's rapid desensitization. Thus, there are numerous theoretically appealing hypotheses for targeting this receptor to improve particularly cognitive functioning in schizophrenia (and in Alzheimer's disease as well).

Future Combination Chemotherapies for Schizophrenia and Other Psychotic Disorders

Given the economic incentives for finding the "cure" and treatment of choice for psychotic disorders, it is not difficult to understand why most drug development activities for the psychoses target a single disease mechanism, with the goal of developing the only therapy for that disorder. In reality, it is probably overly simplistic to conceptualize a disorder with psychotic features as the product of a single disease mechanism. Diseases such as schizophrenia, bipolar disorder, and Alzheimer's disease not only have psychotic features but also a behavioral dimension, a mood dimension, a cognitive dimension, and in some cases a neurodegenerative dimension. It is difficult to conceptualize how such complex disorders could ever be satisfactorily treated with a single entity acting by a single pharmacologic mechanism. For instance, how could a single therapeutic agent for schizophrenia simultaneously treat the positive symptoms of psychosis, the negative symptoms of psychosis, the cognitive symptoms, and the mood symptoms and also prevent further neurodegeneration and repair neurodevelopmental abnormalities?

Perhaps psychopharmacological treatments for psychotic disorders in the future will need to borrow a chapter out of the book of cancer chemotherapy and HIV/AIDS therapy, where the standard of treatment is to use multiple drugs simultaneously to attain therapeutic synergy. Combination chemotherapy for malignancy uses the approach of adding together several independent therapeutic mechanisms. When successful, this results in a total therapeutic response that is greater than the sum of its parts. This approach often has the favorable consequence of simultaneously diminishing total side effects because adverse experiences of multiple drugs are mediated by different pharmacological mechanisms and therefore should not be additive. Clinical trials with multiple therapeutic agents working by several mechanisms can be quite difficult to undertake, but as there is a clinical trial methodology that exists in the cancer chemotherapy and HIV/AIDS literature, this may be an approach that should be applied for complex neurodegenerative disorders such as schizophrenia with multiple underlying disease mechanisms.

Thus, schizophrenia treatments of the future will almost undoubtedly combine an atypical antipsychotic for positive and negative symptoms and for mood, cognition, and hostility without causing EPS, tardive dyskinesia, or hyperprolactinemia with some sort of booster treatment to attain even better relief of negative symptoms (more dopamine?) and cognitive symptoms (alpha-7-nicotinic cholinergic agonist?). Perhaps an additional neuroprotective agent will be helpful if stopping future psychotic episodes alone is not sufficient to arrest the downhill course of illness (perhaps a glutamate antagonist). In the long run, some sort of molecular-based therapy to prevent genetically programmed disease progression or to reverse the consequences of aberrant neurodevelopment may also form part of the portfolio of treatments for schizophrenia.

Summary

This chapter has reviewed the pharmacology of conventional dopamine 2 antagonist antipsychotic drugs as well as the new atypical antipsychotic agents that are largely replacing them in clinical practice. The overlapping features of serotonin 2A–dopamine 2 antagonism of the atypical antipsychotics were discussed, as well as multiple unique features that differentiate each of these agents from each other. Pharmacokinetic considerations for the atypical antipsychotic drugs were reviewed, as were various issues important in the use of these agents in clinical practice. Finally, a wide-ranging view of future therapies for schizophrenia was presented.

Suggested Reading

Andree, T.H., Stack, G., Rosenzweig-Lipson, S., Coupet, J., Marquis, K. WAY-135452, A potent novel D2/D3 partial agonist for the treatment of schizophrenia, Abstracts of the ACNP, Acapulco, Mexico, December 12–16 1999.

Bloom, F.E., and Kupfer, D.J., (Eds.) (1995) *Psychopharmacology: the fourth generation of progress.* New York, Raven Press.

Bond, A.J., and Lader, M.H. (1996) *Understanding drug treatment in mental health care.* Chichester, John Wiley & Sons.

Burris, K.D., Molski, T.F., Ryan, E., Xu, C., Tottori, K., Kikuchi, T., Yocca, F.D. , Molinoff, P.B. Aripiprazole is a high affinity partial agonist at human D2 dopamine receptors, abstracts of CINP, Brussels, July, 2000.

Carey, P.J., Alexander, B., and Liskow, B.I. (1997) *Psychotropic drug handbook.* Washington, DC, American Psychiatric Press, Inc.

Carlsson, A., Waters, N., and Carlson, M.L. (1999) Neurotransmitter interactions in schizophrenia – therapeutic implications. *Biological Psychiatry* **46**, 1388–1395.

Cooper, J.R., Bloom, F.E., and Roth, R.H. (1996) *The biochemical bases of neuropharmacology,* 7th edition, New York, Oxford University Press.

Diagnostic and statistical manual of mental disorders, 4th edition (DSM-IV). (1994). Washington, DC, American Psychiatric Association.

Drummond, J.M. (1997) *Essential Guide to Psychiatric Drugs,* 3rd edition. New York, St. Martin's Press (Paperback).

Dubovsky, S.L. (1998) *Clinical Psychiatry.* Washington, DC, American Psychiatric Press, Inc.

Ekesbo, A., Andren, P.E., Gunne, L.M., Tedroff, J. (1997) (-)-OSU 6162 inhibits levodopa-induced dyskinesias in a monkey model of Parkinson's Disease. *NeuroReport* **8**, 2567–2570.

Feldman, R.S., Myers, J.S., and Quenzer L.F. (1997) *The Principles of Psychopharmacology.* Sunderland, MA, Sinauer Associates Inc.

Frank, E. (2000) *Gender and its effects on psychopathology.* Washington, DC, American Psychiatric Press, Inc.

133

Gelenberg, A.J., and Bassuk, E.L. (1997) *The practitioner's guide to psychoactive drugs,* 4th edition. New York, Plenum Medical Book Co.

Gitlin, M.J. (1990) *The Psychotherapist's guide to psychopharmacology.* New York, The Free Press; Toronto, Collier Macmillan Canada.

Guttmacher, L.B. (1994) *Psychopharmacology and electroconvulsive therapy.* Washington, DC, American Psychiatric Press, Inc.

Hardman, J.G., and Limbird, L.E. (2001) *Goodman and Gilman's The pharmacological bases of therapeutics,* 10th edition, New York, McGraw-Hill.

Hyman, S.E. (1999) Introduction to the complex genetics of mental disorders. *Biological Psychiatry* **45**, 518–21.

Hyman, S.E., Arana, J.W., and Rosenbaum, J.F. (1995) *Handbook of psychiatric drug therapy,* 3rd edition, Boston, Little Brown and Company.

International classification of diseases, 10th edition (ICD-10) classification of mental and behavioral disorders: clinical descriptions and diagnostic guidelines. World Health Organization, Geneva, 1993.

Janicak, P.G. (1999) *Handbook of psychopharmacology.* Philadelphia, Lippincott Williams & Wilkins.

Janicak, P.G., Davis, J.M., Preskorns, S.H., and Ayd, F.J. (1997) *Principles and practice of psychotherapy,* 2nd edition. Baltimore, Williams & Wilkins.

Jenkins, S.C., and Hansen, M.R. (1995) *A pocket reference for psychiatrists,* Second edition. Washington, DC, American Psychiatric Press, Inc.

Jensvold, M.F., Halbreich, U., and Hamilton, J.A. (1996) *Psychopharmacology and women.* Washington, DC, American Psychiatric Press, Inc.

Joffe, R.T., and Calabrese, J.R. (1994) *Anticonvulsants and Mood, Disorders.* New York, Marcel Dekker, Inc.

Kandel, E.R. (1998) A new intellectual framework for psychiatry. *American Journal of Psychiatry* **155**, 457–69.

Kaplan, H.I., Freedman, A.M., and Sadock, B.J. (1995) *Comprehensive textbook of psychiatry,* 6th edition. Baltimore, Williams & Wilkins.

Kaplan, H.I., and Sadock, B.J. (1993) *Pocket Handbook of Psychiatric Drug Treatment.* Baltimore, Williams & Wilkins.

Kaplan, H.I., and Sadock, B.J., and Grebbs, J.A. (1994) *Kaplan and Sadock's Synopsis of Psychiatry.* Baltimore, Williams & Wilkins.

Kapur, S., Zipursky, R., Jones, C., Remington, G., Houle, S.. (2000) Relationship between dopamine D2 occupancy, clinical response, and side effects: a double-blind PET study of first episode schizophrenia. *American Journal of Psychiatry* **157**, 514–20.

Kapur, S., Seeman, P. (2000) Antipsychotic agents differ in how fast they come off the dopamine D2 receptors: implications for atypical antipsychotic action. *J Psychiatry Neurosci* **25**, 161–6.

Kapur, S., and Seeman, P. (2001) Does fast dissociation from the dopamine 2 receptor explain the action of atypical antipsychotics: a new hypothesis. *American Journal of Psychiatry* **158**, 360–369.

Journal of the American Academy of Child and Adolescent Psychiatry, **38**(5) May 1995: Special section: Current knowledge in unmet needs in pediatric psychopharmacology.

Lahti, A.C., Weiler, M.A., Corey, P.K., Lahti, R.A., Carlsson, A., Tamminga, C.A. (1998) Antipsychotic properties of the partial dopamine agonist (-)-3-(3-hydroxyphenyl)-N-n-propylpiperidone (precamol) in schizophrenia. *Biological Psychiatry* **43**, 2 11

Lawler, C.P., Prioleau, C., Lewis, M.M., Mak, C., Jiang, D., Schetz, J.A., Gonzalez, A.M., Sibley, D.R., Mailman, R.B. (1999) Interactions of the novel antipsychotic aripiprazole (OPC-14597) with dopamine and serotonin receptor subtypes. *Neuropsychopharmacology* **20**, 612–27.

Leonard, B.E. (1997) *Fundamentals of psychopharmacology.* Chichester, John Wiley & Sons, Ltd.

Martindale, W. (1996) *The extra pharmacopoeia,* 31st edition, London, Royal Pharmaceutical Society of Great Britain.

Meltzer, H.Y., and Stahl, S.M. (1976) The dopamine hypothesis of schizophrenia: a review. *Schizophrenia Bulletin* **2**(1), 19–76.

Nelson, J.C. (Ed.) (1998) *Geriatric psychopharmacology.* New York, Marcel Dekker, Inc.

Nemeroff, C.B., and Schatzberg, A.F. (1999) *Recognition and treatment of psychiatric disorders: A psychopharmacology handbook for primary care,* Washington, DC, American Psychiatric Press, Inc.

Physician's Desk Reference, 56th edition (2002) Oradell, N.J., Medical Economics Data Production Co.

Pies, R.W. (1998) *Handbook of essential psychopharmacology.* Washington, DC, American Psychiatric Press, Inc.

Prien, R.F., and Robinson, D.S., (eds) (1994) *Clinical evaluation of psychotropic drugs: principles and guidelines.* New York, Raven Press.

Quitkin, F.M., Adams, D.C., Bowden, C.L., Heyer, E.J., Rifkin, A., Sellers, E.M., Tandon, R., and Taylor, B.P. (1998) *Current psychotherapeutic drugs,* 2nd edition. Washiington, DC, American Psychiatric Press, Inc.

Robins, L.N., and Regier D.D. (1991) *Psychiatric disorders in America: the epidemiologic catchment area study.* New York, The Free Press (Macmillan, Inc.)

Sachs, O. (1983) Awakenings, New York, EP Dutton Press.

Schatzburg, A.F., Cole, J.O., and Debattista, C. (1997) *Manual of clinical psychopharmacology,* 3rd edition. Washington, DC, American Psychiatric Press, Inc.

Schatzburg, A.F., and Nemeroff, B. (Eds). (1998) *Textbook of psychopharmacology,* 2nd edition, Washington, DC, American Psychiatric Press, Inc.

Shader, R.I. (1994) *Manual of psychiatric therapeutics.* Boston, Little, Brown & Co.

Siegel, G., Agranoff, B., Albers, R.W., and Molinoff, P. (1999) *Basic neurochemistry: molecular, cellular and medical aspects,* 6th edition. Philadelphia, Lippincott-Raven.

Stahl, S.M. (1997) Awakening from schizophrenia: intramolecular polypharmacy and the atypical antipsychotics. *Journal of Clinical Psychiatry* **58**(9), 381–2.

Stahl, S.M. (1998) What makes an antipsychotic atypical. *Journal of Clinical Psychiatry* **59**(8), 403–4.

Stahl, S.M. (1999) *Psychopharmacology of antipsychotics,* London, Dunitz Press.

Stahl, S.M. (1999) Selecting an atypical antipsychotic by combining clinical experience with guidelines from clinical trials. *Journal of Clinical Psychiatry* **60**(Suppl 10), 31–41.

Stahl, S.M. (1999) Antipsychotic polypharmacy, part 1: therapeutic option or dirty little secret. *Journal of Clinical Psychiatry* **60**(7), 425–6.

Stahl, S.M. (1999) Antipsychotic polypharmacy, part 2: Tips on use and misuse. *Journal of Clinical Psychiatry* **60**(8), 506–7.

Stahl, S.M. (1999) Molecular neurobiology for practicing psychiatrists, part 1: overview of gene activation by neurotransmitters. *Journal of Clinical Psychiatry* **60**(9), 572–3.

Stahl, S.M. (1999) Molecular neurobiology for practicing psychiatrists, part 2: how neurotransmitters activate second messenger systems. *Journal of Clinical Psychiatry* **60**(10), 647–8.

Stahl, S.M. (1999) Molecular neurobiology for practicing psychiatrists, part 3: how second messengers "turn on" genes by activating protein kinases and transcription factors. *Journal of Clinical Psychiatry* **60**(11), 731–2.

Stahl, S.M. (1999) Molecular neurobiology for practicing psychiatrists, part 4: transferring the message of chemical neurotransmission from presynaptic neurotransmission to post-synaptic gene expression. *Journal of Clinical Psychiatry* **60**(12), 813–4.

Stahl, S.M. (2000) Molecular neurobiology for practicing psychiatrists, part 5: how a leucine zipper can turn on genes: immediate early genes activate late gene expression in the brain. *Journal of Clinical Psychiatry* **61**(1), 7–8.

Stahl, S.M., and Shayegan, D. (2000) New discoveries in the development of antipsychotics with novel mechanisms of action: beyond the atypical antipsychotic with serotonin dopamine antagonism. In *Atypical antipsychotics* (MDT), Ellenbroek, B.A. and Cools, A.R. (Eds.). Boston, Birkhauser.

Stahl, S.M. (2001). "Hit and run" actions at dopamine receptors, part 1: possible mechanism of action of atypical antipsychotics. *Journal of Clinical Psychiatry* **62**(9), 670–1.

Stahl, S.M. (2001) "Hit-and-Run" actions at dopamine receptors, part 2: Illustrating fast dissociation from dopamine receptors that typifies atypical antipsychotics. *Journal of Clinical Psychiatry* **62**(10), 747–8.

Stahl, S.M. (2001) Dopamine system stabilizers, aripiprazole, and the next generation of antipsychotics, part 2: illustrating their mechanism of action. *Journal of Clinical Psychiatry* **62**(12), 923–4.

Stahl, S.M. (2001) Dopamine system stabilizers, aripiprazole, and the next generation of antipsychotics, part 1, "Goldilocks" actions at dopamine receptors. *Journal of Clinical Psychiatry* **62**(11), 841–2.

Taylor, D., McConnell, H., McConnell, D., Abel, K., and Kerwin, R. (1999) *The Bethlem and Maudsley NSH Trust. Prescribing Guidelines*, 5th edition. London, Martin Dunitz.

Toru, M., Miura, S., Kudo, Y. (1994) Clinical experiences of OPC-14597, a dopamine autoreceptor agonist, in schizophrenic patients. *Neuropsychopharmacology* **10**, 122S

Vanhatalo, S., and Soinila, S. (1998) The concept of chemical neurotransmission: variations on the theme. *Annals of Medicine* **30**, 151–8.

Van Vliet, B.J., Ronken, E., Tulp, M., Feenstra, R., Druse, C.G., Long, S.K. DU-127090: A highly potent, atypical dopamine receptor ligand – high potency but low efficacy at dopamine D2 receptors in vitro, abstracts of the 13th ECNP Munich, 2000.

Walsh, B.P. (1998) *Child psychopharmacology*. Washington, DC, American Psychiatric Press, Inc.

Zolle, M., Jansson A., Sykova, E., Agnati L.F., and Fuxe, K. (1999) Volume transmission in the CNS and its relevance for neuropsychopharmacology. *Trends in Pharmacological Sciences* **30**, 142–150.

INDEX

Essential Psychopharmacology Continuing Medical Education (CME) Post Test University of California San Diego Department of Psychiatry School of Medicine

ACCME Accreditation

The University of California, San Diego School of Medicine is accredited by the Accreditation Council for Continuing Medical Education (ACCME) to sponsor continuing medical education (CME) programs for physicians. The University of California San Diego School of Medicine designates this continuing medical education activity for 10 hours of Category I credit of the Physicians Recognition Award of the American Psychiatric Association. Each physician should claim only those hours of credit that he/she actually spent on the educational activity.

European CME CNS Accreditation

The European Accreditation Committee for Continuing Medical Education designates this educational activity for up to 10 hours of CME CNS credit points. Partial credit is designated for each unit. Physicians should claim only those hours of credit that he/she actually spent on the educational activity. A 70% pass rate on unit tests is required for successful completion of this activity. Accreditation fee is waived for those physicians wishing to obtain European CNS credit.

Instructions

This CME activity incorporates instructional design to enhance your retention of the didactic information and pharmacological concepts which are being presented. You are advised to go through this program unit by unit, in order, from beginning to end. You will first study the figures and read the figure legends for a single unit of instructional materials, and then go back and read the text that corresponds to that unit, reviewing the figures again as you go. After completing the text, you will then go back over the figures alone for another time. This will allow interaction with the materials, and also provide repeated exposure to the data and concepts presented both visually and in written explanations. Hopefully, this will be fun and interesting, and you will retain new information far more efficiently than you would after just reading the text or listening to a lecture on this topic.

Follow these directions to optimize your learning and retention of "Essential Psychopharmacology".

1. Go through each chapter unit one by one, from beginning to end and in order.
2. View each figure and read each figure legend.
3. Next, read the text while reviewing each figure as you go.
4. Complete the written post-test, using the answer sheet located at the end of the textbook.
5. Review the figures once again, checking any answers of which you are uncertain.
6. Photocopy and fill out the evaluation for the unit you just completed.
7. Fill out the CME registration form.
8. Pay $10 for each category I CME credit you are claiming (up to $100 for 10 credit hours).
9. Send the test answers, evaluations and check for the appropriate amount, payable to "UCSD Department of Psychiatry" to:

   Stephen M. Stahl, M.D., Ph.D.
   5857 Owens Avenue
   Suite 102
   Carlsbad, CA 92009

REGISTRATION FORM FOR CME CREDIT
Essential Psychopharmacology (2nd Edition)
Stephen M. Stahl

Name of Registrant: _____

Address where CME certificate is to be sent::

_____

_____

_____

Number of category I CME credit hours claimed: _____
(CME fee: $10 for each credit hour)

Mail:
1. A check for the appropriate amount made payable to "UCSD, Department of Psychiatry" together with your answers and your evaluations

To:

   Stephen M. Stahl, M.D., Ph.D.
   5857 Owens Avenue
   Suite 102
   Carlsbad, CA 92009

Unit 1: Psychosis and Schizophrenia

Up to 4 Hours of Category I CME Credit

Objectives

1. To review the clinical descriptions of psychosis.

2. To understand the difference between paranoid, disorganized, and depressive psychosis.

3. To discuss the five dimensions of symptoms in schizophrenia, including positive, negative, cognitive, aggressive/hostile, and anxious/depressed symptoms.

4. To review the biological basis of the positive psychotic symptoms.

5. To understand the different functions of the various dopamine pathways in the brain, including the mesolimbic dopamine pathway, the nigrostriatal dopamine pathway, the mesocortical dopamine pathway and the tuberoinfundibular dopamine pathway.

6. To review neurodevelopmental and neurodegenerative hypotheses of schizophrenia.

Self Assessment and Post Test

1. A psychotic disorder is defined as one with delusions, hallucinations, and a thought disorder. True or False.

2. Schizophrenia and drug-induced psychotic disorders require the presence of psychosis as a defining feature of the diagnosis. True or False.

3. Mania, depression, and cognitive disorders like Alzheimer's disease may or may not be associated with psychotic features. True or False.

4. Paranoid psychosis is characterized by severe retardation, apathy and anxious self-punishment and blame. True or False.

5. It is rare for a schizophrenic patient to commit suicide. True or False.

6. Schizophrenia is more common than depression. True or False.

7. The following are characteristic of the negative symptoms of schizophrenia except:
   a. Affective flattening
   b. Alogia
   c. Anhedonia
   d. Acalculia

8. The leading hypothesis for explaining the positive symptoms of psychosis is the overactivity of dopamine in the nigrostriatal dopamine pathway. True or False.

9. Movement disorders are mediated by abnormalities in the mesolimbic dopamine pathway. True or False.

10. The tuberoinfundibular dopamine pathway mediates the secretion of prolactin. True or False.

11. Prolonged blockade of dopamine receptors in the nigrostriatal pathway may lead to an increased sensitization of post-synaptic dopamine 2 receptors and a disorder called:
    a. Parkinsonism
    b. New symptoms of schizophrenia
    c. Tardive dyskinesia
    d. Galactorrhea

12. The severity of which dimension of symptoms in schizophrenia is best correlated with long-term outcome:
    a. Positive symptoms
    b. Cognitive symptoms
    c. Affective symptoms
    d. a and b

13. Cognitive deficits in schizophrenia
    a. Include problems with sustaining and focusing attention, and prioritizing and modulating behaviors based upon social cues
    b. Include problems with verbal fluency and serial learning
    c. Resemble the short-term memory deficits seen in Alzheimer's disease
    d. a and b
    e. All the above

14. A neurodevelopmental etiology for schizophrenia is suggested by all the following except:
    a. Increased incidence in those with obstetric complications in utero
    b. Premorbid and prodromal negative and cognitive symptoms in childhood and adolescence prior to onset of psychotic symptoms
    c. Increased incidence in first-degree relatives
    d. Adult onset of psychotic symptoms with a downhill course during adulthood

15. A neurodegenerative etiology for schizophrenia is suggested by:
    a. Functional and structural abnormalities of brains in schizophrenic patients
    b. A downhill course after onset of psychosis
    c. Less responsiveness to antipsychotic medications the longer treatment is delayed and the more episodes of illness experienced
    d. a and c
    e. All the above

Evaluation

	Strongly Agree	Somewhat in Agreement	Neutral	Somewhat Disagree	Strongly Disagree
1. Overall the unit met my expectations.					
2. My general knowledge about psychosis was enhanced.					
3. The time spent reviewing the five dimensions of clinical symptoms of schizophrenia was just right.					
4. The time spent reviewing the dopamine pathways in the brain was just right.					
5. The time spent reviewing neurodevelopmental and neurodegenerative theories of schizophrenia was just right.					
6. What topics would you like to see deleted or condensed from the unit?					
7. What topics would you like to see added or expanded in the unit?					
8. What is your overall opinion of this unit?					
9. What is your overall opinion of the usefulness of this unit to your practice?					

UNIT 2: ANTIPSYCHOTIC AGENTS

Up to 6 Hours of Category I CME Credit

Objectives

1. To review the pharmacology of conventional antipsychotic treatments: the neuroleptics.

2. To contrast the older conventional antipsychotics with the newer atypical antipsychotics.

3. To review the importance of serotonin 2A antagonism to the atypical clinical properties of atypical antipsychotics.

4. To review the regulatory role of serotonin in each of the four major dopamine pathways.

5. To explain why atypical antipsychotics have fewer extrapyramidal side effects, less tardive dyskinesia, less prolactin elevation, and better improvement of negative and cognitive symptoms of schizophrenia compared to conventional antipsychotics.

6. To review the unique pharmacological properties of several atypical antipsychotics, including olanzapine, risperidone, quetiapine, clozapine, ziprasidone and others.

7. To discuss the pharmacokinetics and drug interactions of atypical antipsychotics.

8. To discuss new drug discovery efforts in schizophrenia, including serotonin dopamine antagonists and other novel agents such as those based upon molecular and neurodevelopmental approaches to drug discovery.

9. To discuss two new theories about dopaminergic modulation of receptors by antipsychotics.

Self Assessment and Post Test

1. The first treatments for schizophrenia were based upon the knowledge that dopamine was hyperactive in the brain. True or False

2. Conventional antipsychotic drugs are also called neuroleptics. True or False.

3. Atypical antipsychotic drugs
   a. Can theoretically block mesolimbic dopamine 2 receptors preferentially, compared to nigrostriatal dopamine 2 receptors
   b. Have selective dopamine 2 antagonist properties whereas conventional antipsychotics have serotonin 2A antagonist properties as well as dopamine 2 antagonist properties.
   c. Have less EPS side effects but also less efficacy for positive symptoms than conventional antipsychotics
   d. None of the above

4. Clozapine is the atypical antipsychotic best documented to improve psychotic symptoms which are resistant to treatment with conventional antipsychotics. True or False.

5. Which of the following serotonin dopamine antagonists (SDAs) is not considered to be a first-line atypical antipsychotic drug?
   a. Risperidone
   b. Quetiapine
   c. Loxapine
   d. Olanzapine

6. The pharmacological property all atypical antipsychotics share is serotonin dopamine antagonism. True or False.

7. The new atypical antipsychotics including risperidone, olanzapine, and quetiapine act by:
   a. Blocking dopamine-2 receptors
   b. Blocking serotonin-2 receptors
   c. Both of the above
   d. None of the above

8. The ratio between the blockade of serotonin receptors and dopamine receptors differs for various classes of antipsychotic drugs. True or False.

9. The interaction between dopamine and serotonin in the nigrostriatal dopamine pathway may explain why serotonin dopamine antagonists have propensity for reducing extrapyramidal reactions. True or False.

10. Which pharmacologic properties in addition to serotonin 2A/dopamine 2 antagonism characterize one or more atypical antipsychotics?
    a. Dopamine 1, 3, and 4 antagonism
    b. Serotonin 1D, 3, 6, and 7 antagonism
    c. Serotonin and norepinephrine reuptake blockade
    d. Alpha 1, alpha 2, muscarinic and histaminic receptor blockade
    e. All of the above

11. Which atypical antipsychotics are substrates for CYP450 1A2?
    a. Clozapine
    b. Olanzapine
    c. Risperidone
    d. a and b
    e. All the above

12. Which atypical antipsychotics are substrates for CYP450 2D6?
    a. Risperidone
    b. Clozapine
    c. Olanzapine
    d. All of the above

13. Smoking could lower clozapine and olanzapine plasma levels. True or False.

14. Molecular approaches to the treatment of schizophrenia attempt to identify an abnormal gene product in order to compensate for this abnormality. True or False.

15. Treatment of schizophrenia in the future may involve the combinations of various mechanisms of action simultaneously. True or False.

16. Conventional antipsychotics may cause EPS because they bind tightly to D2 receptors and thus prevent any dopamine from being able to bind to those receptors. True or False.

17. Dopamine system stabilizers are partial agonists, increasing levels of dopamine when they are too low and reducing dopamine levels when they are too high. True or False.

Evaluation

	Strongly Agree	Somewhat in Agreement	Neutral	Somewhat Disagree	Strongly Disagree
1. Overall the unit met my expectations.					
2. My general knowledge about serotonin regulation of dopamine was enhanced.					
3. The time spent reviewing conventional neuroleptic drugs was just right.					
4. The time spent reviewing the class of atypical antipsychotics was just right.					
5. The time spent reviewing individual atypical antipsychotic drugs was just right.					
6. What topics would you like to see deleted or condensed from this unit?					
7. What topics would you like to see added or expanded in this unit?					
8. What is your overall opinion of this unit?					
9. What is your overall opinion of the usefulness of this unit to your practice?					